The Ultimate Male Solution

- Lose the Belly
- Increase Testosterone
- Supercharge Your Sex Life

By Brad King

D1441354

Table of Contents

Part III

Introduction

I can't believe almost three years has passed since I wrote *Beer Belly Blues*. For those of you who aren't aware, *Beer Belly Blues* was an award-winning bestselling book I wrote on the syndrome almost every man eventually experiences. It's been referred to by a number of different names including male menopause, man-o-pause, andropause, viropause or, as most women like to call it, The Grumpy Old Man Syndrome. Given the last moniker, one would be left to believe that such a syndrome only afflicts the very old – that would be a very wrong assumption.

The fact is, many men experience a decline in their male hormones – primarily the manliest of the manly male hormones, testosterone – after the tender age of 30. If you are one of the lucky ones who have been able to keep your youthful vigor and physique right into your 40s, well the Male Menopause Syndrome will eventually bite you in the ass as well – just give it time.

I coined the phrase the "Beer Belly Blues" for two specific reasons: **1)** because it is more often than not associated with a bigger waistline, and no man is going to openly admit that he is getting fat. However he will admit that drinking beer is a manly thing to do (thus the beer belly) and, **2)** most men will also experience various grumpy dispositions or full-out depression (thus the blues), followed by a general lack of a zest for life. Quite simply, men who experience a precipitous drop in their testosterone have a very difficult time losing body fat – primarily from the abdominal area – and an all-too-easy time accumulating it. Aside from this, healthy testosterone levels are imperative for keeping a man healthy and happy. The equation goes something like this: higher testosterone = greater neurochemical production = enhanced motivation and extra uplifting mood chemicals.

What almost every man needs to come to terms with is the fact that he is not going to look great in a Speedo® much past his thirties. Now I'm not condoning the wearing of such a bathing apparatus at the best of times, but suffice it to say that some of us dudes look pretty darn good in the things whether you want to admit it or not! The problem is that as men lose their testosterone, they lose their once toned, muscular bod, and from there everything goes south – literally!

It turns out that testosterone may be the most important health factor in the male body. When it is naturally abundant, it's at the very core of everything we hold sacred as men – especially our never-say-quit libidos, not to mention our penchant for getting an erection at the most awkward of times. It's also behind our incredible energy and stamina and, of course, our confidence. But as we inch past the 30-year mark and start to realize that we are passing our prime, testosterone starts saying *adios* and we begin to experience fatigue, fat accumulation, low moods, cardiovascular and blood sugar problems, a loss of sexual interest and a keen interest in a new class of prescription meds designed to help get it up and keep it there long enough for sex!

When I first wrote *Beer Belly Blues* I had a rough idea of how many men needed the information within that book. What I didn't know was how that information would really impact their lives. Since releasing that book, I have had countless men approach me at various seminars and health shows just to say thank you for what the information within those pages helped them overcome. The other thing that I had no way of knowing at the time was how many women were going to embrace that book and, in turn, thank me over and over again for impacting their lives in such a positive way because, as one woman put it, "My man is back!"

The *Ultimate Male Solution* came about because of the sheer number of men that asked if I could put all of that incredible information with *Beer Belly Blues* into practice and design a manual of sorts. The *Ultimate Male Solution* is a means for men to not only learn about the various conditions associated with the Beer Belly Blues, but a practical guide that shows every man exactly how to eat, exercise and supplement for optimal testosterone production. Aside from these vital areas, men will also learn what to ask their health professionals about testing for various hormones and blood markers, in order to assess their continual progress.

Men wanted a book that would guide them on a path to a better way of looking, feeling, performing and even thinking. Well here it is. No more excuses! Time to get your hairy butt off the couch and make things happen. If you still have plenty of testosterone to go around, power to you. This book will help protect your levels and ensure that you are around to enjoy them for a long time to come. But, if you are already experiencing some of what you will learn in the coming pages, or are well into the Beer Belly Blues, this book will help get you back to the place you once were, or at least the place you always wanted to be.

Come on, you've always wanted to be the ultimate male. Well you've finally found the solution – *The Ultimate Male Solution*!

Part I

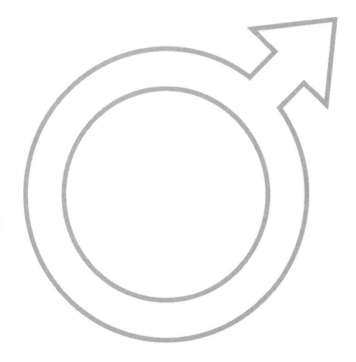

Chapter One:
The Male Transition

The side table is littered with balled-up tissues. A half-empty bag of potato chips is spilling onto the coffee table. Slightly dented beer cans are strewn haphazardly around a frantically spinning fan. You know you should get up and do something ... go to the gym maybe, or at least clean the place up ... but you have no energy, and it all makes you feel so sad. You just want to eat and not think about the fact that you don't even want to get laid. There can only be one answer to "What the hell happened in here?"

You are going through man-o-pause.

Known technically as "andropause," this is your version of that frightening grandma lore, the "Great Change." Some like to refer to it as male menopause – though with no meno to pause, this doesn't really make sense. I simply call it as the Beer Belly Blues for the very reason that this not-so-kind transition is more often than not associated with a larger-than-life belly and a mood more akin to a woman who's been wronged one time too many! Hey, women don't call it the Grumpy Old Man Syndrome for nothing.

The fact is if you're like the majority of men over the age of 30 living on planet earth, it may already be upon you. That's right. By the time that "third decade's a charm" thing comes around, your dreams of being Superman may be waning and, as you will soon find out, you may actually be transitioning a little closer to a Lois Lane then any man would care to admit. Can you say "Estrogen Dominant?"

Blame testosterone. This primary male hormone is the culprit behind the Beer Belly Blues. When abundant – like it is in your teenage years and throughout your twenties when you actually carried a six pack in your middle instead of your arms, and when you couldn't control that thing between your legs, and you slept through the night instead of getting up multiple times to stand over the bowl waiting for what seemed an eternity for a few drops to emerge – testosterone fills you with vigor and a sex drive that won't quit. It gives you your muscles, a metabolism that allows you to eat copious amounts of pizza and Twinkies without becoming fat, and a libido that was perpetually taking applications for new friends. Right around your thirtieth birthday, however – and most definitely by the time you enter your forties – the amount of testosterone in your body begins its slide downhill. In fact, as I pointed out in my bestselling book *Beer Belly Blues*, us men can easily lose 10 percent of our testosterone levels each decade after age 30, and by the time we are 60 we typically produce 60 percent less testosterone than we did at age 20. Yikes!

And if for some reason you think the Beer Belly Blues is for all those other poor saps and has somehow passed you over, think again. A blood analysis of nearly **8,000** men aged **30-70** showed shocking percentages of testosterone deficiency. It turns out that only **4.2 percent** of men had optimal testosterone levels even though the great majority of these men would otherwise be considered healthy … or at least thought they were.

As the testosterone in your body diminishes you will begin expanding and decreasing in all the wrong places. No longer will you have a lean body or boundless energy, and your engine might need a little bit of a jump start to get going. The Beer Belly Blues (andropause) is marked by several symptoms including decreased energy, lowered metabolism, lessened muscle mass, thought and memory issues, anemia, increased body fat (once again, enter the beer belly), diminished sex drive or sexual ability, and depressed mood (ah, yes, those inevitable blues). A reduction in testosterone is also linked to increased risk of cardiovascular disease and diabetes.

Basically, the Arithmetic Table of Testosterone would read something like this:

Adequate levels of testosterone = dopamine production (a feel-good brain chemical) + motivation + muscles + sex + an all-around happy dude

OR

Diminished testosterone = you are one flabby, weak and miserable person to be around.

Which would you choose if you had the choice? The great news is you do have a choice!

No need to completely lose hope, give in to the depression, whip out your harmonica and start playing the Beer Belly Blues just yet. Noticing the physical and emotional effects of reduced testosterone does not have to be a hopeless situation. Rise Andropause Army! Stare diminished testosterone down and take back your life. Age may take our testosterone, but it will not take our manhood … at least if I have anything to say about it! This book will give you the tools you need to live a disease-free life of abundant health, energy and vitality – one in which you don't have to rely on little blue pills in order to get blood flowing in the right direction again! And maybe, just maybe, get you into that Superman suit yet.

We can work on the rally cry as we move through. So, what are you waiting for? Follow me…. .

Chapter Two:
Your Life on Testosterone

Quick quiz: *It's 10 o'clock on a Friday night. What are you doing?*

Just getting ready for a night out with the boys? Maybe if you are in your twenties. If you have slid into your thirties, and especially if the big 4-0 has come your way, the answer might sound a little more like "lying on the couch and making my belly a table for a can of beer while I watch TV."

The thing is, when men hit their 30s and testosterone begins to diminish, so does their zest for life. The Beer Belly Blues steals more than just your muscles and ability to think clearly when playing that rousing game of Scrabble your wife decided it would be fun to organize with the neighbors every week. Andropause can also take away quality of life, and even years from it.

Other studies have shown that men dealing with the Beer Belly Blues face many issues that detract from their quality *and* quantity of life. You may notice that you don't have the energy you once did, the sexual vigor or the brain power. Where you once faced each day with a take-no-prisoners zip you may find yourself feeling a little down in the dumps, or perhaps just plain "blah." That is the testosterone – or lack thereof – talking.

This overall sense of disinterest isn't the only thing that *hypogonadism* (the fancy scientific term for diminished testosterone, particularly during andropause) can cause. Studies have demonstrated a drastic spike in the mortality rates of men with low testosterone. Compared to men with normal testosterone, those living with the Beer Belly Blues (i.e. diminished testosterone) experience **88 percent** higher mortality rates. And, no, those statistics are not bloated by men who throw themselves off of cliffs when they realize – or don't – that their testosterone is dropping.

The Beer Belly Blues are sort of like running the gauntlet … just without the cool battle scars to later show off. Experts have developed two scales to evaluate the effects of diminished testosterone on the lives of men going through the Beer Belly Blues. Known as the Aging Males' Symptoms scale, and the Age-Related Hormone Deficiency-Dependent

Quality of Life scale – or the AMS and A-RHDQoL, respectively – they are used to explore the relative effect of the reduction of testosterone on men's quality of life.

If it depresses you that you are facing a time in your life with scales that have been reduced to acronyms, it might help to remember other fixtures in your life such as CNN and ESPN. Acronyms are your friend. Just keep telling yourself that.

These scales have identified seven areas that are affected by the Beer Belly Blues. Conveniently, each of these areas is also a major part of quality of life. And so you run the gauntlet. These areas are:

- Physical functioning
- Social functioning
- Social-emotional functioning
- Mental functioning
- Energy
- Emotional functioning
- Sexual functioning

All of your favorites, right? Well, these scales weren't created for the purpose of illustrating why the world should implement mandatory euthanasia at the age of 32. Despite the discomfort that is often associated with these topics and the unwillingness to discuss them, those men who are willing to put a voice to the ideas of the Beer Belly Blues are helping others understand andropause. And with understanding comes the ability to rise above it. Remember our battle cry? That's right. Something *can* be done about dwindling testosterone, and it doesn't require chemicals or anything drastic. You really can get your life back, and I'm going to show you how in the coming pages – promise!

First, though, let's take a hard look at what testosterone means to your energy, your belly, your muscles, your brain, your heart, your blood sugar, your unit and your prostate. The more information you have, the more likely you are to take up the battle cry!

Chapter Three:

////////////// **Your Energy on Testosterone**

Your whole life isn't centered in your pants. Ok, well maybe it is a little bit. Testosterone does a lot more than getting your little swimmers going and your muscles bulging. When the Beer Belly Blues claims you, you will start to notice that it's not just your little swimmers moving along that you are concerned about. Sometimes it's just having enough energy to get out of the bathtub before you need to hook yourself up to scuba equipment.

Testosterone is responsible for a lot of things in your body, including your metabolism (i.e. the rate at which you are able to convert food into energy). When you hit the Beer Belly Blues and your testosterone diminishes, your metabolism may feel like it's coming to a screeching halt. This is due to the fact that healthy testosterone levels are needed for your body to process what you eat efficiently. When your metabolism was working at its peak, like it did during the Golden Age of your teens and twenties, the food that you ate was quickly converted to energy. Your body then burned this energy before it could be turned into fat. This is what keeps you from getting fat even if you can put competitive eaters to shame. When your testosterone began slipping away, your metabolism declined along with it. A slow metabolism will not convert your food quickly, which means that you won't get the same energy out of food and you will begin to feel the effects of energy-deficit (as in, "Help me, I have no energy!").

When your metabolism slows you will notice two fun symptoms: your body will spread and your energy will drop. And as we all know, when your energy drops, your body spreads some more. Your body will start clinging to all the fat that it possibly can. This fat will then make you feel even less energetic, so you won't feel like exercising. Not exercising will add on even more fat, and the spiral begins (I will discuss this in more detail in the next chapter).

During the Beer Belly Blues your body will also reduce its production of red blood cells. Red blood cells are responsible for carrying oxygen throughout the body to the various systems, and then carrying away the waste products. This action keeps your body feeling refreshed, and your systems operating at peak efficiency. When your body does not produce as many of these useful little oxygen transporters, it sometimes leads to the condition referred to as *anemia*. Aside from the fact that your organs and muscles can't get as much oxygen as they require, leading to weakness and fatigue, anemia can also lead to:

- Irritability
- Shortness of breath
- Headaches
- Sore tongue and bleeding gums
- Nausea and loss of appetite
- Faintness and dizziness
- Confusion and dementia
- Increased heart rate

Oxygen is what fuels every cell within your body, so a lack of it will throw a cog in your metabolic machinery, thereby causing almost every cell in your body to be sluggish (this includes your immune system, heart, muscles and brain, all of which require copious amounts of oxygen to continue to function at peak efficiency).

Research out of Queens University in Ontario, Canada, has shown that anemia can actually be treated through testosterone replacement therapy in certain cases. This makes total sense when you consider that testosterone is required for the stimulation of *erythropoietin* (a protein that regulates red blood-cell production) as well as the percentage of the concentration of red blood cells in the body (referred to as *hematocrit*).

Needless to say, reduced red blood cells will leave you feeling weak, drained and decidedly floppy. Add this to your body's new aversion to metabolizing anything and you are left gaining unwanted body fat just by thinking of your mom's famous crême brulée. As an added cruel joke, the Beer Belly Blues also comes with erratic sleep patterns and frequent insomnia. Even if you used to be one of those men who could comfortably snooze through the apocalypse, you may find yourself tossing, turning and counting through multiple generations of sheep every night, which, of course, leads to reduced energy and increased body fat … and reduced energy and increased body fat … and reduced energy, etc.

Sleep Your Way To Higher Testosterone

Loss of sleep is actually one of the most detrimental things to experience where a man's testosterone status is concerned. All hormones work in a cyclical fashion and testosterone is no exception. Testosterone levels peak in the early morning (around 8 A.M.) and decline throughout the day (hitting a low around 8 P.M.). Research indicates that those who experience deeper (uninterrupted) sleep patterns, also experience higher testosterone levels.

One study from the University of Chicago discovered that quality sleep is one of the best ways to predict morning testosterone levels in older men. Another study from the University of Montréal in Quebec, Canada, revealed that men with low testosterone experience a loss of "deep sleep" (referred to as phases III and IV). When we are young – say in our 20s – we tend to spend a lot more time in "deep sleep" (10-20 percent of total sleep), compared to when we reach middle age and beyond. It's no wonder, since youth is also synonymous with high testosterone levels! By age 50, men begin to spend between 5-7 percent of their sleep time in "deep sleep." After that, it's all downhill. Studies show that by age 60, "deep sleep" is almost nonexistent – right along with an older man's testosterone levels.

Decreased energy is among the most common complaints that men have as they age. A drop in energy also leads to many of the other problems associated with the Beer Belly Blues, including social disinterest, lack of motivation and decreased overall quality of life. Aside from understanding these key symptoms, there are various lab tests (which I discuss in the last section of this book) that can accurately diagnose low testosterone and the accompanying reduced red blood-cell production. On average, your testosterone will decrease by about 1 percent every year after you turn 30. Some guys are able to skim by for a few years before Operation Testosterone Drop begins, and others somehow end up the target of much more sudden decreases. Either way you will eventually start noticing that the spring in your step is decidedly less springy, and that your belly seems to be picking up the slack.

It is a leading theory that men who had particularly high testosterone when they were younger are more likely to notice the effects of the Beer Belly Blues, even if their testosterone remains at the same level as other men experiencing the syndrome. This is because men with high testosterone tend to be thrill seekers who have higher energy, more sex drive and the tendency to participate in behaviors such as abusing controlled substances. When these men experience the dip in testosterone associated with the Beer Belly Blues the lethargy and disinterest, as well as the social and sexual effects, are more devastating.

You don't want to waste your life being a lethargic blob. Reclaiming your energy is not out of your reach. Experts say that efforts to increase testosterone can make a huge impact on your energy level, and give you back that zest for life you've been so desperately craving.

Chapter Four:
////////////////// **Your Belly on Testosterone**

Have you ever caught yourself walking past the maternity section in the clothing store and coveting those pants with the stretchy bands on the top? If you nodded yes, you are probably experiencing ... well, I think you get the picture by now. When you consider that the rapid expansion of the belly is one of the most common complaints a man experiences once he ends his twenty-something years, it's no wonder that I dubbed this transitional period the Beer Belly Blues.

Though there has been some debate over the actual biological cause for decreasing testosterone in aging men, it has become accepted that the Beer Belly Blues is already present in men beginning in their thirties, and that this reduction in androgens (another fancy term for sex hormones, i.e. testosterone) contributes to many physiological and psychological symptoms.

There is the loss of lean muscle mass, along with an increase in body fat. This is due to many factors, most of which are not fully understood. Don't let those somewhat frightening pictures of Joe Pilates in his tights deceive you. No matter what your wife's fitness instructor tells her, most men will not have washboard abs and bulging arms when they are ninety. It just doesn't happen ... well, unless you have the genes of Jack Lalanne! What does happen is that testosterone evacuates the premises when you get past age thirty and your body starts a slow decline into a squishy place. For some this decline is slower than for others. And for those others it can seem like you went to bed one night wearing the same pajama pants you've had since college (after many trashcan rescues and convincing your adoring other half that the flannel and haphazard stitches will stand up for another season), and the next day you were staring longingly at the maternity pants.

The reason andropause is referred to as the Beer Belly Blues as opposed to just the Overall Chubby Blues is that the decrease in overall testosterone in a man's system during this period is directly related to the increase in both subcutaneous fat (the fat that is close to the surface, right under the skin, that gives one an appearance of being overweight) as well as visceral fat (also known as organ fat or intra-abdominal fat, located deeper in the body and packed in between the internal organs).

More specifically, men experiencing testosterone deficiency are more subject to the rapid gain of fat around the middle (aka the birth of the Beer Belly). Studies have indicated a direct correlation between testosterone deficiency and a man's waist circumference (see box below). This is due to the fact that the relationship between testosterone levels and weight is specifically applicable to abdominal obesity and not obesity in general.

Low testosterone has been linked to excess belly fat for many years. But it wasn't until the last decade or so that studies started confirming this theory. Norwegian researchers were the first ones to actually discover that most men can determine whether they are deficient in testosterone simply by looking at the size of their waist. The researchers discovered that men with waist sizes greater than 40 inches were experiencing on average 30 percent lower testosterone levels than men with waist sizes that were 37 inches or less.

Don't start thinking that it is your beloved box of Twinkies that is the enemy and that you will never again be able to indulge in the creamy goodness without becoming disturbingly creamy yourself. It is not simply that low levels of whole-body testosterone are responsible for an increase in body fat. When it comes to the Beer Belly Blues, the times they are a' changing. Not only will your body cling to body fat like nobody's business, but also its overall composition will be altered. Instead of a tendency toward a composition dominated by lean muscle mass and bone, your body will shift to a composition featuring a larger percentage of adipose tissue. Adipose tissue is the soft, hard-to-cast-away version of body fat that is not immediately translated into energy. And if you happen to be a fan of British science fiction you know that while adipose can be an adorable villain, it is also what makes you round around the middle.

This adipose is particularly fond of colonizing your abdominal region, developing into a beer belly even if you have sworn off your weekly six-pack. As usual, blame testosterone, or more appropriately, the lack thereof. Fortunately, this correlation also has its converse association. Do you remember the Vicious Cycle? Well, there is a cycle here, too. It has been demonstrated that men with higher body weights tend to have lower testosterone, and that men with lower body weights tend to have higher testosterone. This can be explained in that men with lower testosterone tend to be tangled in the grips of the Beer Belly Blues and, therefore, are experiencing a simultaneous increase in body fat and decrease in testosterone.

The correlation can be approached in another way as well. While men in the midst of the Beer Belly Blues may be fighting like a teenage girl near swimsuit season to get the pounds off, it has been shown that the men who are able to decrease their weight can also increase their testosterone (as long as that weight comes from stored fat and not muscle). Simultaneously, those who can increase their testosterone may experience weight loss. Here enters the cycle. If your weight goes down, your testosterone goes up. If your testosterone goes up, your weight goes down. And so on and so forth.

Italian researchers have discovered that testosterone is able to positively influence the fate of your fat cells by:

- inhibiting the fat cells' ability to expand by taking in fewer lipids
- inhibiting *lipoprotein-lipase* (a powerful fat-storing enzyme)
- stimulating *lipolysis* (fat break down) by increasing the number of *lipolytic beta-adrenergic receptors* (fat-cell membrane receptors responsible for the release of stored fat).

After reviewing numerous efficacious studies (placebo-controlled) of testosterone therapy on aging men, Australian researchers discovered that the majority of the men receiving testosterone supplementation also experienced significant decreases in body-fat levels with increases in lean body mass. Not surprisingly, the men who experienced the greatest effects (lowest body fat and most muscle mass) were the ones with the lowest starting levels of testosterone.

And as it pertains to your growing beer belly, it is important to understand that a bulbous belly doesn't just bring you closer to the Pillsbury Doughboy Effect and put a damper on your sexy factor. A study done by Johns Hopkins University highlighted the dangerous correlation between central adipose tissue (belly flab) and cardiovascular disease. Belly fat puts a lot of pressure on all of your internal organs, but particularly on your heart. This makes your heart have to work extra hard to get the blood pumping through your body, and can lead to heart disease and a higher instance of heart attacks. This doesn't mean that the next time you step on your bathroom scale and notice that the little arrow ticks up a few extra spots that you need to clutch your heart and commit yourself to bed rest. Weight is just one of the factors that increase your risk of heart disease. Two measurements are taken into consideration when calculating increased cardiovascular risk, your BMI

(Body Mass Index) and your hip-to-waist ratio (I'll talk more about what testosterone means for your heart a little bit later).

The hip-to-waist ratio is used during many of the studies. This ratio, in case you are a little shaky on where all your more obscure body parts are, is the comparison of the measurement around your belly and the measurement around your hips – regardless of how big around you are anywhere else. This ratio is one reason why a man who weighs 300 pounds but looks like he was forged from steel is considered healthier than a 170-pound man of the same height that sports a testament to the Beer Belly Blues.

By now you may be realizing that the Beer Belly Blues are like a big web that constantly turns back on itself. The symptoms of decreased testosterone aren't fun enough on their own; they have to contribute to each other. I've talked a little bit about the Beer Belly Blues and the jiggly bod that comes along with it, but what you might not realize is that the reduction of lean muscle mass directly contributes to the growth of your belly bulge. This is because lean muscle tissue burns more calories than does a comparable mass of fat. When your body composition changes to favor adipose tissue instead of muscle tissue, it loses a lot of its ability to burn calories.

Want another equation from the Arithmetic of Testosterone?

A sluggish metabolism + reduced muscle tissue + increased adipose $= $ **Beer Belly**.

But would I tell you all of this if you were doomed to a life of never being able to hula hoop again for fear of getting stuck? In the coming pages I will let you in on some of the best ways to increase your testosterone and fight off the beer belly in the process.

Chapter Five:

////////////////// **Your Muscles on Testosterone**

Imagine you are strolling down a hall when you see a mirror in front of you. You stop and strike a few poses, admiring the slim, muscle-bound body reflected back at you. Feeling pumped, you move on to the mirror hanging beside it and notice that reflected you is decidedly less impressive. Your muscles aren't exactly qualifying you for the next super-hero calendar shoot and you are looking a little saggy in your midsection.

Welcome to the Beer Belly Blues House of Mirrors! That first mirror is the you that you remember from your twenties, the one you've secured into your brain as what you will always look like. Unfortunately, the second mirror is captioned "Reality Check." This mirror reminds you of the cruel, dark truth behind the Beer Belly Blues.

So, you're already on to testosterone's sick little game of making a quick escape during your thirties and into your later years, and how this leads to the energy of a slug, a protruding belly and a loss of your spark for life. Brace yourself. Now it's time to talk about your muscles.

Don't get me wrong … I know that back in the day you could lift heavy things and take off your shirt on the beach without fear of rebellion from fellow sunbathers, even when you wore that dreaded Speedo® (yes, the one you still have buried deep in your bottom drawer). The problem is, when the Beer Belly Blues hit, things start to go wrong where your muscles are concerned. Aging doesn't just cause a lack of energy and reduced metabolic rate. The natural – or unnatural, depending upon how you view it – process of getting older creates changes in the actual structure of a man's body. Your organs and bodily systems will start to function less efficiently, as every cell within your body functions better when testosterone levels are in the healthy range.

This is where our Vicious Cycle returns yet again. When the structures of your body begin to change as a result of aging and diminishing testosterone production, numerous problems begin to emerge. One of the most noted structural changes that occur during the Beer Belly Blues is the reduction of muscle tone and strength.

Secondary effects of decreased testosterone such as flagging energy are partially to blame for your muscles functioning like they have been run through the tenderizer. This is due to the fact that when you have less energy you are less likely to continue working out or participating in other physical activities that encourage the development and maintenance of muscle tone.

This slow slide toward a life dominated by hammocks and big-screen TVs cannot take the full rap for your loss of muscle strength and mass, though. Muscles are a system like the cardiovascular or nervous system, and are likewise subject to independent structural change during the Beer Belly Blues. To understand this we should go back to the Beer Belly Blues House of Mirrors.

Look back in that first mirror and admire your toned, developed physique. If you harbor the deep, dark secret that you dream of being a world-class bodybuilder, feel free to slather your imaginary self with baby oil and channel your inner Arnold Schwarzenegger. I'll give you a few minutes ...

All right, back to the discussion at hand. In that mirror you were overflowing with testosterone. This testosterone contributed to the strength and mass of your muscles by aiding a process called "protein synthesis." This synthesis is the process by which your body takes the proteins you eat and uses their amino acids (the building blocks of protein) to rebuild, repair and renew existing strictures such as your various muscles. These amino acids are used like tiny little Lego blocks to ensure the muscles that comprise your musculoskeletal system have what they need in order for you to remain buff. Other muscles, such as your heart and smooth muscles, are created using other processes, but all are dependant upon amino acids as their primary building blocks. In otherwords, you are one big muscle – or at least you used to be!

Testosterone not only aids in the building of muscles, but it also prevents atrophy and helps your muscles resist fatigue during activity. You may have noticed by now that testosterone is the ultimate multi-tasker. When it comes to your muscles testosterone functions like building a motorcycle, fueling it and oiling its parts all at the same time.

Now step back over to the second mirror. Take a moment to wipe off the baby oil and get dressed as you mourn the loss of your muscles. In this mirror your body has lost much of its testosterone. This has made a major change to the overall composition of your body, including a shift toward lower muscle tone. Protein synthesis is still limping along, but without the flood of testosterone to help it your muscles aren't being built as quickly.

This isn't just a problem because your muscles won't be growing. When protein synthesis drops, so does the ability of your muscles to maintain their current condition.

Performing any type of physical activity, from walking to lifting weights to doing the electric slide at your cousin's wedding, causes your muscles to break down microscopically. In young bodies, this breakdown leads to your muscles coming back bigger, stronger (the theme from *Rocky* is playing over and over in my head as I write this), and ready for action. Without testosterone aiding protein synthesis, your muscles won't be able to keep up and you will become a smaller, flabbier and weaker version of your former self.

Instead of your muscles grabbing onto the protein from that steak you put away for dinner and using it to rebuild your worked muscles, the process is only partially effective. Some of that protein will go toward supporting your muscles, while much of that steak just gets detoured to your burgeoning beer belly. This means that your muscles don't get the chance to build back up and so they gradually they lose their tone and strength. Don't think that you can combat this by moving in to the gym and spending your downtime hooked up to a constant stream of protein shakes. If you don't want to relinquish your muscles to the Beer Belly Blues you have to get to the root of the problem … all together, now … TESTOSTERONE.

The Metabolic Engine

The amount of muscle we carry dictates how many calories we are able to burn each day (referred to as our resting metabolic rate). The problem is, with age comes a decline in lean muscle mass followed by a reduced metabolism. In order to maintain an efficient metabolism after age 35, it is imperative to ensure adequate protein intake, with special emphasis on three amino acids – leucine, isoleucine, and valine – referred to as the branched-chain amino acids or BCAAs (which comprise over 35 percent of the essential amino acids in muscle tissue) due to their unique branch-like shapes.

Research presented in the *Journal of Nutrition* showed that by adding proteins (approximately 125 grams/day) known for their high amounts of BCAAs, people were able to maintain muscle mass while reducing body fat during weight loss. The study looked at protein foods that provided optimal levels of the branched-chain amino acid, leucine. Dr. Donald Layman, professor of nutrition at the University of Illinois where the study was conducted said, "Traditionally, people have built a diet around low-fat foods instead of high-quality protein foods. Study participants following the moderately high protein plan were twice as effective in maintaining lean muscle mass."

Don't you worry about your shrunken little body just yet, as I will discuss ways to easily raise your BCAA levels throughout the day, and help you restore your muscles to youthful grandeur in Part III.

Increasing your levels of testosterone will give the protein-synthesis process a boost and your muscles will be on their way towards new growth and recovery. Now, I'm not promising that you will be able to once again march around in that lime green Speedo® you should have thrown out years ago, and star in the Beer Belly Blues Bodybuilding competition (however, if you want to, more power to you, but you might find yourself a little lacking in participants). But taking a few simple steps toward increasing your natural sex hormone levels will protect your muscles and help keep you going strong.

Let's go back to the House of Mirrors one more time and stand in front of the You in Your 20s mirror. Burn that image into your mind because it may just be making reappearance in the near future.

Stay with me. You really don't have to settle for kissing your muscles goodbye when the heydays of your twenties wind to a close. I promise in the coming pages that I will show you ways to increase your testosterone naturally, and reclaim your muscle tone and strength in the process.

Chapter Six:
Your Brain on Testosterone

By now you've probably caught on to the basic idea behind the Beer Belly Blues. Of course, if you haven't it would be totally understandable considering that another fantastically fun symptom of the Beer Belly Blues is, in official BBB Army terms, a broken brain.

To be a little more scientific, the Beer Belly Blues is marked by psychological symptoms including depression, as well as functional symptoms. These functional symptoms include memory loss, difficulty processing information, even an increased instance of Alzheimer's disease. So next time your main squeeze accuses you of slipping into senility, feel free to wave your hands around and babble incoherently at her for a few minutes before flipping to Part III of this book and finding out what you can do about your squishy brain matching your squishy body.

Before you find out how raising your natural testosterone levels acts like a repair kit and energizer all-in-one for your brain, let's talk a bit about what's going on in the first place. Don't forget what our brave hero GI Joe taught us: Knowing is half the battle. GI Joe! Go Joe! (Duke would *never* have had the Beer Belly Blues!)

Grumpy Old Man Syndrome

If you asked most women if they had a name for a man's midlife transition, they'd probably say "the Grumpy Old Man Syndrome" before you could finish the question. The problem is, they'd be right, but then again, when aren't they?

According to myriad research, testosterone has a remarkable ability to lift a man's spirits and make him come alive again. Among its many seemingly miraculous attributes, testosterone is a great antidepressant. According to a study appearing in the *Journal of Clinical and Experimental Endocrinology and Metabolism* that included 856 men aged 50 to 89, depression rates were elevated in nearly direct proportion to falling testosterone levels. The older the subjects tested, the lower their testosterone levels and the higher the incidence of depression. Interestingly, 25 men in the study were already being treated for clinical depression and were on prescription antidepressants. All 25 of these men were found to have the lowest testosterone levels of the entire group – on average 17 percent lower.

In an Australian study of nearly 4,000 older men, which appeared in the journal *Archives of General Psychiatry*, researchers revealed a strong link between low testosterone and depression. The study revealed that men who suffered from depression experienced significantly lower testosterone levels than men who had no symptoms of depression. In fact, men with abnormally low testosterone are on average 271 percent more likely to show clinically significant signs of depression than men with higher testosterone levels.

Although it is not known exactly how testosterone enhances mood and reduces depression, it is believed that it works by enhancing a feel-good brain chemical – one that is often low in those suffering from low motivation and depression – called dopamine. Another theory is that testosterone aids mood by enhancing energy levels in the brain, and throughout the entire body. Testosterone is actually essential to healthy energy production. In fact, many of the enzymes that manufacture high-energy compounds to run our bodies greatly depend upon adequate testosterone for their own production. And finally, there's always that sexy uplifting feeling (called ego) a man derives from his muscularity and strength, all of which require gobs of testosterone to maintain as we age.

According to numerous researchers, the Androgen Deficiency in Aging Males (ADAM) questionnaire is highly effective when screening for low testosterone levels. Our friend ADAM asks a series of delightfully prying questions and uses your responses to make an educated guess about your testosterone levels. Many of these questions deal with your thought processes, memory and how you have been feeling emotionally. Though it was originally designed as a study to determine if the prevalence of certain groups of symptoms are more common in men with decreased levels of testosterone, the ADAM questionnaire has been accepted as a way to detect insufficient testosterone once men hit 40. If you've hit the big 4-0, embarking on a little getting-to-know-myself quest with ADAM may be a good start in the battle with the Beer Belly Blues.

It's important to remember that testosterone levels are not static throughout your twenties and then make a sudden drop. Your sex hormones will fluctuate during your life. These temporary dips, even if they are relatively large such as those documented in the first few months of being a father, don't affect cognition. Rather, it is consistently diminished levels during the Beer Belly Blues years that can make it difficult for you to finish that Sudoku puzzle and accidentally call your wife by your college ex-sweetheart's name – either way, you're in trouble!

Studies have also indicated that being over 40 makes a man's brain particularly vulnerable to the effects of low testosterone. Though decreased testosterone can have other ill-effects on younger men, the Endocrine Society suggests that the status of a man's sex hormones don't have any real measurable effect on brain functioning when he is young, but it can make a major difference in protecting his brain as he climbs over the hill and slides down the other side.

Feeling a little sad and foggy isn't the only risk to your brain during the Beer Belly Blues. A study of 547 men between the ages of 59 and 89 performed by the Department of Family and Preventative Medicine at the University of California was conducted to investigate whether levels of testosterone and cognitive functioning can be used to predict each other. Participants were put through a battery of tests during which many of them probably pretended that they were in training for the CIA. These included category fluency tests, function evaluations, and Visual Reproduction recall tests.

Despite assumptions otherwise, results were shown to be independent of factors including BMI, education, cigarette or alcohol use, and age. The performance on the various tests could be grouped only in terms of the amount of bioavailable testosterone in the participant's system. Through these tests it was determined that higher sex hormones are directly related to superior cognitive performance (think of your brain on steroids). This was especially true for the memory tests. It seems that memory attempts to cling to testosterone and all the happy thoughts of youth, slipping away as your levels drop.

It isn't just your inability to recall what you ate the day before, or the fact that your daily exercise regime may begin to consist primarily of walking into the same room several times without any idea of why you are there that may be cause for concern during the Beer Belly Blues. Other studies looking at the implications of various sex hormone levels indicate that significantly decreased testosterone in aging predisposes men to memory deficit disorders such as Dementia and even Alzheimer's disease.

Though it is not entirely understood how a lack of testosterone increases ones risk for memory disorders, it is assumed that like other systems and structures within the body, the brain undergoes functional changes – many of which are less than desirable – during the Beer Belly Blues. In terms of testosterone, The Oxford Project to Investigate Memory and Aging performed by the University Department of Pharmacology and the Radcliffe Infirmary Trust in the United Kingdom suggests that testosterone protects structures in the brain – primarily the hippocampus – that are responsible for memory and emotions. When hippocampal neurons begin to wear out or become damaged, various emotional disorders and memory problems begin to emerge. If the damage is severe enough, then full-blown conditions such as Dementia and Alzheimer's disease can arise. By studying the relative severity of Dementia-related symptoms in association with the level of testosterone in study participants, Oxford theorized that decreased androgens – in which testosterone is the primary one – can contribute to the decline of *neuroplasticity* (Quite a word, right? It just means the ability of the little neurons in your brain to be flexible in response to what is going on around you. Think Silly Putty.) and neuronal loss.

Neuroplasticity

It wasn't that long ago when neuroscientists believed that your brain structure is fixed or unchangeable once it has fully developed after childhood. However, new research is showing that numerous aspects of the brain remain plastic or changeable throughout our lives. This ability for the brain to change both structurally and functionally because of environmental cues is referred to as neuroplasticity or brain plasticity. Neuroplasticity allows the brain to reorganize and adjust itself in order to compensate for injury and disease or for learning and new activities.

This study was a direct follow-up to a previous investigation of the impact of overall testosterone levels on cognitive testing performance. It seems that United Kingdom testosterone has the same effect as North American testosterone – the study showed that regardless of age, controlled-substance use and BMI, lower levels of testosterone led to less-than-stellar performance on cognitive tests.

And for those of you who are conspiracy theorists, this study was performed on two different levels. Aging men with low testosterone levels were observed and tested for indications of Dementia and Alzheimer's disease, but to ensure that the results were not being misconstrued, patients that had been diagnosed with Alzheimer's disease through independent evaluations were also screened for testosterone deficiency. From both angles, decreased sex hormones were shown to be a factor in the development and severity of Dementia and Alzheimer's disease.

All right, take a few deep breaths. I know that was a lot of heavy information for your testosterone-starved brain. All is not lost. You don't have to go find a baby blue bathrobe and begin eating only puréed food in preparation of being committed to Old Folks' Layaway. There are ways to get your testosterone back up to fighting form so it keeps protecting all your neurons for years to come. In coming chapters I will give you the tools you need to increase your testosterone naturally and get your brain back.

Chapter Seven:
////////////// **Your Heart on Testosterone**

Hearts are not just the cute shape full of chocolate that you buy for Valentine's Day. Whether it's manly to admit it or not, you have one and it isn't pointy on the bottom with two curves at the top. In fact, your heart is a rather ugly-looking muscle that beats – on average 90,000 times each day – in order to propel oxygen-infused blood through nearly 100 thousand miles of blood vessels, some of which (called capillaries) are barely wider than the blood cells they are transporting. And despite it looking like a primeval sea creature, your heart is actually pretty vulnerable. Many things, from diet to lifestyle to various physiological factors, can lead to heart damage and disease. This is a real bummer because without a functional heart, life goes downhill pretty quickly.

Now that you have gotten comfortable with the Beer Belly Blues, I have another condition to throw at you: *metabolic syndrome*. Don't worry, there isn't going to be a quiz. This is just another part of this point in your life that will make you look back fondly on that period in your mid-twenties when your friends said you were going through a "Quarter-Life Crisis" because you got your ear pierced twice, started a reggae band, bought a beachcomber and started spending your evenings writing melodramatic poetry. Ah, those were the days.

Metabolic syndrome is described by the ADAM (remember our friend from the brain chapter? Oh, well, maybe you don't …) Medical Encyclopedia as being "a group of risk factors that occur together and increase the risk for coronary artery disease, stroke and type 2 diabetes." Though research has not been able to pinpoint an individual cause for the condition, several risk factors have been identified. As you may have guessed, these factors closely mimic those of the Beer Belly Blues. The strongest risk factors for developing metabolic syndrome are:

- Central obesity – remember the squishy, protruding belly that earned the Beer Belly portion of the Beer Belly Blues moniker?

- The body's inability to utilize insulin effectively to process blood sugar – known as insulin resistance.

Other risk factors, which should also seem familiar, include:

- Hormonal changes
- Lack of exercise
- Aging

The American Heart Association in cooperation with the National Heart, Lung, and Blood Institute has recently emphasized the impact of metabolic syndrome on aging men's health. You may have metabolic syndrome if you have noticed three or more of these indicators:

- High blood sugar as can be determined by fasting levels
- Large waist measurements
- Low HDL cholesterol (the good kind!)

What matters about all of this is that when you are going through the Beer Belly Blues, metabolic syndrome can greatly increase your odds of heart disease and damage. Some believe that this syndrome, and its components, is to blame for decreases in bioavailable testosterone, while others argue that it is the reduction of testosterone that leads to the risk factors of metabolic syndrome.

It is not just this ambiguous syndrome that makes traversing the Beer Belly Blues akin to your heart dancing through a minefield. Research conducted by the Department of Medicine at Columbia University College of Physicians and Surgeons indicated that dramatic alterations in sex hormones, particularly a consistent dip in testosterone, may be an underlying factor not only in the contributing risk factors of cardiovascular disease, but in the disease itself.

Studies suggest that reduced testosterone is associated with hypertension, cardiac failure and ischemic heart disease, which is marked by reduced blood supply to the heart muscle. A relationship has been identified between testosterone deficiency and the overall function of the heart. Inflammatory responses and the reactivity of the smooth muscles within the vascular system are negatively affected by an interruption in the balance of sex hormones. This leads to reduced function of the heart muscle, and the overall cardiovascular system.

Was that confusing and medical enough for you? Good. Now I'll talk about testosterone's place in the life of your heart. Bear with me as I use the Beer Belly Blues Army lingo.

Think of metabolic syndrome as a conglomeration of factors that band together to increase your risk of such fun conditions as heart disease and stroke. While it may seem like this is just a catch-all term that was created by confused researchers who just wanted to blame something and get home to their evening pot roast, metabolic syndrome is a real condition that has been able to link various health factors. By understanding the metabolic syndrome, researchers have been able to better study the correlation between causes, symptoms and larger health concerns. This combines with the other complaints of the Beer Belly Blues, such as reduced energy, poor metabolism and an alteration in body composition to favor adipose tissue over lean muscle mass – all of which put your heart right in the danger zone.

Like just about everything else in your body, your heart is part of a larger system that depends on a variety of factors to operate properly. Let's go back to that motorcycle we talked about last chapter. Your heart trying to function without the cooperation of the other parts of the system is like just the engine of a motorcycle thinking that it will get anywhere without the body and wheels. It may have all of the juice, but it won't get very far if it doesn't have the rest of the machinery to help it along.

When it comes to your heart, the rest of the machinery includes arteries and veins. To work well these blood vessels have to have optimum conditions. Unfortunately, when the Beer Belly Blues hits, your blood pressure tends to spike and, along with increasing levels of inflammation, triglycerides and LDL (bad cholesterol), your blood highway starts to clog up. Think of this like a faulty fuel line. If the blood from your heart can't get through the vessels to the rest of your body, your other systems start to suffer. This leads to your heart working extra hard to keep things working. And as we all know, working too hard is bound to cause problems.

Beyond just the blood vessels that act like a monorail system getting blood to and from your heart, your heart muscle itself is vulnerable to damage and disease when the Beer Belly Blues start sucking away your testosterone. Testosterone helps the smooth muscles of your heart react appropriately to various degrees of stress and activity. When your testosterone levels drop, these reactions become dulled and the muscle can't respond as well. Not only does this mean that day-to-day functioning is diminished, but the risk of heart disease increases, as does the instance of sudden heart failure. That would be enough to just about ruin anyone's day – make that life!

Don't think that this is the chapter in which I tell you to give up, start browsing the organ transplant list, and seriously consider that Viking funeral that you conjured up in your college years. Like all other aspects of the Beer Belly Blues, the risk of cardiovascular problems can be dramatically reduced with the increase of available testosterone. In the coming pages, I will share with you some ways that you can improve your natural levels of testosterone.

Chapter Eight:

////////////////////// **Your Blood Sugar on Testosterone**

Type 2 diabetes has gotten a lot of attention recently as its prevalence rapidly increases. While we might not see a bunch of children dressed as little diabetes monsters this Halloween, the condition is a scary enough threat for many people. While factors such as obesity, poor diet and genetic predisposition put a large portion of the population at risk for developing type 2 diabetes, the Beer Belly Blues gives us "aging" men the special distinction of being right at the front of the line.

Aside from this, testosterone also plays an important role in helping insulin do its job effectively. The reason this is so important is because insulin happens to be the premier fat-storage hormone of the body (more on this in Part II) and excess levels of it (*hyperinsulinemia*) are directly connected to how much fat you are able to store. The problem is that hyperinsulinemia is almost always associated with a condition known as insulin resistance, wherein the body's cells become resistant to insulin and thereby summon even more insulin into the blood. In fact, the majority of men who experience insulin resistance (which leads to type 2 diabetes) are known to suffer from low testosterone levels.

The correlation between low testosterone and type 2 diabetes is so established that British researchers at Barnsley Hospital in the UK discovered that at least 40 percent of men with type 2 diabetes had low testosterone levels, while other studies show an even greater correlation. For instance, researchers from Johns Hopkins School of Medicine in Baltimore have estimated that up to 64 percent of men who suffer from diabetes exhibit diminished levels of testosterone. Regardless of what the true percentage is, the connection is undeniable.

It probably doesn't come as a surprise that your Body Mass Index (you may have heard your doctor say something about your BMI) has a strong correlation with your risk for developing type 2 diabetes. BMI is a measurement that was developed as a way to measure one's risk of disease from being overweight – although it has nothing to do with the real issue at hand, which is how much actual body fat are you carrying. Even though it does not actually give an accurate measure of percentage of body fat, it gives a good idea of your overall body composition. This measurement uses your height and weight to group you into categories from "underweight" to "obese." Within these categories there are further classifications that specify the degree to which you fit into the category.

For example: Three men that are each 6' 3" weigh 210, 310, and 350 pounds. According to the World Health Association (WHO), they are all in the "obese" range, but they are classified as mildly obese, moderately obese, and severely obese, respectively.

BMI has lost appeal as an accurate way to determine the health of an individual, but is still widely used to evaluate impact on the health of large groups. You may be wondering why any of this matters. Well, here it comes.

A study reported in *Diabetes* indicated a correlation between BMI and insulin, but also between a decrease in the effectiveness of insulin and – *drum roll, please* – lower testosterone levels.

Insulin and glucose are what are responsible for the development of type 2 diabetes. If you think that women in the midst of a chocolate craving are fussy, meet your body and its blood sugar levels. The human body is incredibly delicate when it comes to blood sugar. It wants the levels to be kept within an inflexible window or it starts getting angry, and it uses the pancreas to keep blood sugar behaving properly. When glucose (read: sugar) levels dip too low, the pancreas releases glucagon that tells the liver to release extra glucose. If the levels get up too high, the pancreas starts churning out insulin that recruits fat cells to suck some of the glucose out of the blood. Either way, normal blood sugar levels are achieved, and everything is good again.

Issues start to arise when your body starts to protest against this process. Research has shown that both BMI and testosterone levels have a serious impact on the effectiveness of insulin on glucose. When your body becomes – as the all-powerful "they" call it – *insulin resistant*, your blood sugar spikes. If this goes on without being put back in check, type 2 diabetes rears its ugly head.

The problem is that most aging individuals experience a rise in blood sugar levels and exaggerated blood sugar levels eventually lead to conditions like *hyperinsulinemia* (constantly elevated insulin levels) and when the islet cells (the cells responsible for producing insulin) eventually wear out, full blown type 2 diabetes. Blood sugar levels are usually measured by a fasting blood-glucose test, whereby a patient is expected to fast for anywhere between eight and ten hours prior to having his/her blood drawn. This is to allow for enough of a time period where blood sugar can be at its lowest value in the bloodstream. Even though much of the medical community recognizes **126 mg/dL** as the fasting glucose threshold for a diagnosis of diabetes, newer research shows that the optimal fasting blood glucose levels should always be between **70–85 mg/dL**. When men allow their levels to rise past **85** (mg/dL), they experience a **40-percent** increased risk of death from cardiovascular disease.

This is where the Beer Belly Blues comes in. Unless you are planning on entering the Guinness Book of World Records for late-life growth spurts, your BMI will increase along with your weight. This means that when your muscle mass begins to surrender and the body fat moves in, your BMI will go up and cooperation between your blood sugar with insulin will start to drop. The correlation between BMI and blood sugar is particularly important when it comes to the Beer Belly Blues because not all fat is created equal. Though any form of obesity is a breeding ground for disobedient blood sugar, visceral adipose tissue (squishy belly fat) has a more significant link to insulin resistance.

Body fat is not just responsible for your BMI creeping up. Important research has recently pointed to the double-edged sword relationship between body fat and sex hormones. It has long been understood that fat behaves as a highly effect manipulator of hormones. Especially as you get older your fat tissue starts getting in touch with its feminine side by secreting an enzyme known as *aromatase* that takes testosterone and turns it into a powerful form of estrogen (which I will be covering in Part II). This means that your testosterone levels go down and the Beer Belly Blues begin with a vengeance.

The other side of the sword comes with the understanding that while excess belly fat leads to decreased testosterone, decreased testosterone leads to increased fat (you may remember the Vicious Cycle from the discussion of the beer belly). This has led to the strong recommendation that men experiencing an increase of weight during the Beer Belly Blues should do everything in their power to lose the beer belly in order to help raise testosterone levels naturally (I'll show you how to achieve this in Part III). Catching testosterone at the beginning of the downward spiral can mean preventing the development of type 2 diabetes later down the line.

As mentioned earlier, older men who have developed type 2 diabetes have a higher tendency of diminished testosterone. This is related to the body's decreased ability to dispose of excess glucose when its testosterone levels are low. While this is useful information because those who have developed type 2 diabetes can undergo testing for diminished testosterone levels in order to head more ill-effects of low sex hormones off at the pass, it can also be used in reverse.

As men get older and the Beer Belly Blues looms in the not-so-far distance, keeping track of their testosterone levels can help them monitor their risk of developing type 2 diabetes.

This understanding whips me right back around to metabolic syndrome. Remember how metabolic syndrome gives you an achy-breaky heart? The cardiovascular risk is only a part of this syndrome. The contributing factors, particularly central obesity, also combine to wreak havoc on your blood sugar.

These associations were first identified through careful examination of men undergoing treatments for prostate cancer. These treatments, known as "androgen deprivation therapy," purposely decrease a man's testosterone levels in order to combat cancer in the prostate. I'll talk more about testosterone and your prostate a bit later. This information matters now because this intentional decrease in testosterone levels caused a flood of largely unexpected side effects.

More than half of the patients who were being treated with androgen deprivation experienced a notable increase in central obesity, decreased response to insulin and elevated blood glucose levels. Realizing this inspired researchers to look at testosterone-related studies from a different angle. They noticed that in the same way that men who were sacrificing their testosterone for the good of their prostates showed vulnerability toward metabolic syndrome and its minions, when testosterone was increased the progression of metabolic syndrome was stalled and blood sugar began to respond to insulin more normally – hello-o-o-o-o.

Some of the more innovative researchers are now encouraging men to undergo serum testosterone screening as a part of their regular health-maintenance routine. You can fit it in right between taking your Flinstone's gummy vitamin (please know that was a joke) and running three laps around the bathtub during your shower (that, not so much a joke). Keeping a heads-up on your testosterone levels is like doing guerilla warfare on type 2 diabetes. When you know that decreased androgen levels are its secret weapon, you can pull a sneak attack by boosting your testosterone.

Don't worry if your strategy skills dulled before you could conquer Germany in *Risk*. I'll outline a battle plan in coming chapters. And never fear, you aren't doomed to a life of grilled tofu (actually, I don't ever recommend soy or soy-related products), broccoli and water. Bidding a fond farewell to your three glazed doughnut breakfast of champions may be a good first step toward keeping your blood sugar in check, but you will soon find out that you can still live a perfectly normal life while increasing your testosterone and keeping diabetes at bay.

Chapter Nine:
////////////////// **Your Unit on Testosterone**

Consider, for a moment, the history of rock 'n' roll, in particular how the contributions of a single member can elevate the greatness of the whole. Can you imagine Led Zeppelin without the thunderous drumming of John Bonham, or a version of KISS without the stage presence of Gene Simmons? Who would Van Halen be without the frantic fretwork of Eddie Van Halen (aside from a band with a high probability of a different name)?

The same rings true for all sorts of music, and the Beer Belly Blues are no exception. The star of this show? The male organ – please hold your applause till the end (what did you think I was going to tell you to hold?).

Unfortunately, the quality of our "instrumentation" ages less like The Beatles than The Monkees. We become more likely to be afflicted by conditions such as late onset hypogonadism (aka the Beer Belly Blues), suffering from a range of symptoms such as a decline in sexual interest, inability to climax and the dreaded ED – erectile dysfunction. As the saying goes; *erectile dysfunction is nature's way of saying no hard feelings!* OUCH!!!

Unlike our helpful friend ADAM from Chapter 6, there really is no upside to ED (pun intended). I'm sure by this point you've been around long enough to hear that old axiom beginning, 'It's not the size of the boat…," right? Let's just put it this way; whether you spent your younger years fancying yourself a luxury cruise liner or a dependable little tug boat, ED is that guy who makes sure your ride will be much closer to a half-deflated life raft.

As terrifying as that may sound, the outlook is considerably brighter. Interest in the study of both the causes of and solutions for erectile dysfunction has blossomed over the last few years thanks to a few aging male researchers who didn't exactly like what they were beginning to experience and the emergence of several effective oral therapies and the population growth within the most heavily affected age demographics. In fact, a recent international survey found no fewer than 23 independent international studies hard at work on the case.

For instance, a recent study in Vienna surveyed 2,869 men between the ages of 20 and 80 in order to investigate the strength of the correlation between several potential risk factors and the presence of erectile dysfunction. After examining a wide list of criteria such as BMI, tobacco usage, alcohol usage and cholesterol, they concluded the factor most significantly tied to ED was age. While by now this may not surprise you, the degree to which this is true is jaw dropping, as the risk for ED as much as doubled when transitioning from one age bracket to the next.

However, as we all know, age is just a number, and it isn't the year printed on the calendar that is threatening to keep our Jolly Rogers at half-mast. A similar study, conducted with 675 participants between the ages of 45 and 60, sought to test the link between ED, testosterone levels (specifically low serum total testosterone and low serum bioavailable testosterone) and BMI (which we touched briefly on in Chapter 8). Researchers observed that for each year of age added, there was a comparable decrease in the International Index of Erectile Function score (indicating a greater risk of ED). As this progression ran parallel with the decrease in levels of both forms of testosterone, it suggests a shared interrelationship amongst the three. Furthermore, the most severe cases of ED were up to three times more likely to be experienced by individuals with low testosterone.

Testosterone and Erections

The relationship between testosterone and a healthy erection has been scientifically documented. Testosterone is a well known promoter of nitric oxide (NO), which is required for optimal blood flow (restricted blood flow is one of the reasons behind erectile dysfunction). Testosterone is responsible for stimulating nitric oxide within the expandable erectile tissues, called the corpora cavernosa. Research presented in the *Journal of Sexual Medicine* indicates that aside from its powerful arousal qualities, testosterone can also improve erectile function by restoring the blood-trapping capacity of blood vessels within the penis. The same journal presented a study showing that testosterone therapy was even more effective when combined with the erectile dysfunction drug, sildenafil citrate (Viagra®).

The effects, like a woman's ideal relationship, are not purely physical, however. Although scientists have still yet to definitively prove the role testosterone plays in maintaining one's ability to go "full steam ahead," one must also remain conscious of the mental aspect involved in effectively captaining the HMS Proper Unit Function. To remain with the boat theme, think of it this way: even the finest canoe carved from the mightiest tree is, if lacking the paddles of inspiration, just another piece of hollow wood (hey, you try thinking of a better analogy).

The Massachusetts Male Aging Study (MMAS) suggested that lower testosterone levels led to a decrease not only in erectile function, but also in overall libido as well. Or, more simply, it takes more than the equipment itself being functional to get the job done. After all, jackhammers don't fix sidewalks and ruin my night's sleep all by themselves. They take a dedicated operator, ready and willing to put their tool to use. However, the findings of the MMAS suggest some of us may be nearing retirement in more ways than one, as they discovered a "sharp decrease in sexual activity with old age."

How sharp? A mere eleven-year age differential meant up to a 47 percent drop in subjects who reported themselves as being sexually active. A good bit of this might be attributed to a simple matter of desire, as indicated by the statistics of a follow-up study that probed the category of "thinking about sex." About 40 percent of men in their 40s reported that they thought about sex 'every day,' compared to only 12 percent of men in their 70s. Were this not enough, an astonishing eighteen times as many men in the latter group claimed to think about sex "never or less than once a month" as did men in the former. Hmmm, I wonder what the stats would be for guys in their 20s?

Whether it is a matter of technical difficulty or operator error, a dysfunctional unit can be a matter of great anxiety. But rest assured that it isn't just you (or me, or THAT GUY SNEAKING UP RIGHT BEHIND YOU RIGHT NOW! … Just kidding. Got your mind off that serious stuff for a second though, didn't I?]). It's an issue so important to so many people that we have some of the best minds massaging it (sorry, couldn't resist), making progress even as we speak. And the answer doesn't reside in some blue pill shaped like a diamond. In fact, I'll be discussing some of the pitfalls associated with ED drugs in Part II.

What is important to keep in mind is that issues such as ED are hardly anything to be embarrassed or self-conscious about. Aging is something we cannot stop, nor should we want to, for with age comes wisdom and maturity, not to mention potty training and diapers, and I can guarantee you issues of that sort would be much harder to explain to anyone you're lucky enough to bring home for the evening.

See? Things could be much worse. I can feel you cheering up already. And in the coming pages I will tell you how to get things … looking up. Hope you can rise to the challenge (once again, sorry)

Chapter Ten:

/////////////////// **Your Prostate on Testosterone**

In terms of how often you think about different parts of your own anatomy in the course of everyday life, your prostate ranks somewhere between your appendix and your anal sphincter in popularity – although your anal sphincter is the trap door that allows Dr. Probe access to your prostate in the first place. To review, the prostate is a walnut-sized gland located between the rectum and the bladder that surrounds the urethra like a donut. Though it is chronically overlooked and underappreciated (no thanks to all the other exciting bits in the neighborhood), that's not to say it doesn't perform an important function. The prostate gland, in fact, plays a key role in the success of reproductive chemistry, as it contributes to the fluid that comprises a man's ejaculate fluid, including a chemical that causes the female genital tract to contract, thus helping to transport sperm toward the uterus through the fallopian tubes. The amazing part is that the prostate gland just happens to achieve all this while keeping what might be considered a low profile.

Think of it this way: if, as we discussed in the last chapter, your unit is the lead singer or the virtuoso guitarist, your prostate is the bass player who stands in the background and loads the gear into the van while the rest of his band-mates party. Were it not for all those doctors that left us singing a slightly higher-pitched version of the Beer Belly Blues, we might forget we had one altogether. This would be problematic, to put it lightly, as those examinations aren't just some insidious plot by the rubber-glove cartel to boost profits.

One of the things they are rooting around for down there is *prostatitis*, an inflammation of the prostate gland most commonly attributed to infection. This mild condition is often treated by prostate massage, as this process assists in ridding the body of harmful bacteria. By the way, don't even think about calling up your local Massages-R-Us Center and asking if they perform this kind of massage. Trust me, it never goes well.

A slightly more serious condition that is tested for is *benign prostatic hyperplasia*, or BPH, otherwise known as an enlarged prostate. This is a condition encountered with increased frequency beginning around the age of 30 and escalating along with the age of the patient. Its symptoms include a range of urinary problems, such as retention, an irritating sensation while urinating, bladder pain, and a heightened risk of urinary tract infection. While these issues are hardly insignificant, they are fully manageable via a combination of scientifically validated nutrients – that will be discussed in Part II – and a few minor adjustments to your habits. Steps as simple as limiting highly processed foods, trans fats, alcohol and caffeine intake and making sure to take regular bathroom breaks to alleviate discomfort will get your mind out of your pants in no time.

The real source for consternation (triple word score!), however, is the big C-word. Although prostate cancer is the second most common cancer in men – not to mention the number-two cancer killer of men in the civilized world after colon cancer – scientists have yet to determine its exact cause. What is known, however, is that the risk of developing it increases in conjunction with increased age, as shown by a recent study involving individuals who had died of other causes. Subjects showed evidence of prostate cancer in up to 30 percent of cases involving individuals in their 50s, and an astonishing 80 percent of those in their 70s – a statistical leap that is not only significant, but is certainly tough to dismiss, especially when considering the manner in which testosterone levels naturally decrease with age.

The survival rate for men diagnosed with prostate cancer within five years of initial onset is very high, nearing 100 percent. But beyond five years, if the cancer has spread to other organs, the survival rate drops to 38 percent. According to recent cancer statistics, prostate cancer is now being diagnosed in men at the same rate as breast cancer in women.

While it has yet to be scientifically proven, the suggestion here is that these diminishing levels of testosterone affect the prostate in a negative fashion, as it is heavily dependent upon androgens, particularly **dihydrotestosterone** or DHT, for the regulation of its function. In a sample of 77 men with a low total testosterone or free testosterone levels, Harvard researchers found what they described to be a "high prevalence of biopsy-detectable prostate cancer." Also convinced in the possibility of a link between the two, scientists at the Memorial Sloan-Kettering Cancer Center in New York pursued a study of the potential correlation between low testosterone levels and post-cancer surgery prostate health.

The PSA Test – Is It All That?

Prostate-specific antigen (PSA) is a specialized protein produced by prostate cells. When the prostate swells, PSA is produced by virtue of the presence of a larger surface of the organ. Prostate disorders can also cause leakage of PSA into the blood stream, which is why a PSA test may or may not be an indicator of the presence of disease. Unfortunately the PSA test has one of the highest error rates of any medical test today, often misdiagnosing patients. For every six biopsies ordered because of a PSA reading, only one cancer is discovered. According to a leading urology journal most men who score high on the PSA test turn out not to have cancer at all, just an elevated level of PSA.

Despite problems with the test, urologists believe that when a PSA score returns very high, the chances of the presence of cancer go up, since cancer causes the most PSA to be present in the blood as compared to a simple non-disease prostate enlargement. So what is normal? An index score **1.0** is considered normal, while any reading over **4.0** is considered cause for concern. Just as concerning is the upward movement of the score over a short period of time, even if that score remains below **4.0**. If your score doubles from **1.0** to **2.0** within a year, start paying attention, even though you are well below the **4.0** threshold.

The reason behind the intrusive rubber-glove exam – the doctor is feeling the prostate itself for firmness, which in conjunction with the PSA test is a better indicator of potential disease – is that neither it nor the PSA test is definitive. Only a biopsy – surgical extraction of tissue from the prostate for lab testing – can return a definitive diagnosis, however a second and even third opinion is always a smart choice before allowing a piece of you to be removed and examined, no matter how small that piece may be.

Fortunately, the situation isn't as grim as it may seem. Prostate cancer is frequently described as a slow-growing cancer, and while this is not always the case, more often than not this means that treatment can begin before the disease becomes too advanced. A wide variety of detection methods, including the aforementioned physical examination (i.e. finger probe) and prostate-specific antigen (PSA) testing, afford doctors the chance to identify the cancer at the earliest stage possible and take action to stop it from spreading.

While standard practices for treatment include radiation therapy or surgery, more severe cases might be met with stronger measures such as chemotherapy, cryotherapy or anti-androgen/estrogen therapy (these drugs are the equivalent of castrating a man). Continued testing by medical professionals is being conducted in hopes to procure even more effective methods of dealings with prostate cancer, despite a lack of funding and general public awareness in comparison to certain other similarly pervasive forms of cancer. However, perhaps the most important diagnostic tool is closer than you might think.

Unfortunately, most of the traditional treatments for prostate cancer and other forms – especially radiation therapy and chemotherapy – don't always attack cancer cells specifically, and thereby often cause harm to otherwise healthy cells that surrounding the tumor. For instance, radiation therapy forms ions as it passes through the body (which is why it is referred to as ionizing radiation) and these ions have the ability to damage the genetic material (DNA) inside the cells. In fact, DNA damage is the first stage in the creation of cancer. Chemotherapy drugs are just as problematic – if not more so – as radiation therapy due to the massive creation of cell-destroying molecules known as *free radicals*. It is the excessive free radicals that are produced as a byproduct of chemotherapy that causes damage to healthy tissue. Some chemo drugs cannot be continued or used in the first place because of this disastrous side effect.

There isn't a synthetic compound or a fancy piece of equipment in the world that could replace one's own sense of self-awareness in monitoring and ensuring one's health, even pertaining to a malady seemingly as intimidating as prostate cancer. After all, at the end of the say we are all our own responsibility and no one can save us but us. We can take control of our destiny by doing everything we can to keep an eye out for indicators that something is wrong. Some warning signs to look out for include pain in the bones (especially the ribs, spine, pelvis and femur – or, as I like to call it, the crotch-to-knee bone), as well as weakness of the legs, trouble urinating (delayed stream, leaking/dribbling, straining) and incontinence. However, these issues don't always manifest themselves until the later stages, if at all. This makes it increasingly important to remain vigilant even in the absence of obvious symptoms, which in turn is where once again those wonderful doctor visits come in.

To not maintain a regular schedule of check-ups to ensure the health of your prostate simply because "everything feels all right" would be akin not worrying if a grenade rolled in through your front door simply because the pin was still in it. You would hardly consider it safe just because it hadn't exploded yet, would you? The same goes for your prostate, at least figuratively speaking. The explosion might be less spectacular, but the damage remains absolutely real. In 2005 alone, the United States saw 30,000 deaths due to prostate cancer in addition to approximately 230,000 new diagnoses.

As unpleasant and inconvenient as it may seem, keeping on top of your prostate health is a top priority. The great news is that there are also a class of nutrients that are highly beneficial when it comes to prostate health and prostate cancer prevention and … you guessed it … I'll be covering these in Part II.

Part II

The Truth Shall Set You Free

All right, Beer Belly Blues Army, how's our morale doing? Not great? That's understandable considering all of the problems I have just told you about. But bear with me. I told you there was no need to pack it in, purchase that cemetery plot (or draw up your will to ensure your family will comply with your desires for a traditional Viking funeral), and check yourself into the nearest retirement village to feed birds and wait for the end.

I promised you I would tell you all about ways you can boost your testosterone without resorting to dangerous and largely ineffective chemicals, and take charge of your life. Well, I'm about to get closer to making good on my promise.

In this section I am going to lay it all out for you. You're going to learn more about your body and why we need to care about all of the different elements that go into making it function properly. I'll also talk to you about your diet – no, no, don't put the book down! I'm still not going to tell you that you are now restricted to one aisle of the grocery store and that it will all contain things that you are used to scraping off of the bottom of your boat or feeding to that Easter bunny your little girl just had to have last Spring. I'm talking real food for the real world – and some myths about food that may surprise you.

And speaking of myths, how often have you thought about falling victim to one of those commercials featuring a couple that looks way too happy to be dancing in the kitchen while making dinner, and then suddenly disappears into their bedroom? Have you ever picked up the phone to call that "confidential" toll-free number so that you could start popping pills in the hopes of raising your testosterone – or your unit? A lot of men have. But I'm going to tell you why you need to change the channel when those commercials come on – or at least why you should chuck something close by at the TV (your wife does call those throw pillows doesn't she?) while declaring "You can't have me! I won't submit!"

All right, perhaps that is a little dramatic, but you get the point. I'm going to fill you in on why these pharmaceuticals are far from the best option when trying to cope with decreasing testosterone or your limp …

personality. And, yes, I'll fill you in on the ways that you really can get yourself back on track. We'll talk supplements and a highly effective form of "really short duration" exercise, and slide ever closer to your marching orders in Part III when I sketch out your plan for charging headlong into a more productive and satisfying middle age.

Rise Beer Belly Blues Army! It's time to fight!

Chapter Eleven:
Not All Testosterone is Created Equal

Over the last few chapters, we discussed the effects of testosterone on different anatomical systems (I know, you're probably still stuck on how testosterone affects your unit), and what you might expect as you advance through the Beer Belly Blues. Now it's time to turn our attention to testosterone itself for just a minute.

While by now you have enough knowledge on the subject to make you dangerous, the details of what goes on behind the curtain might still be a bit hazy, sort of like all the little parts that go into your car. It's one thing to be able to list things like the radiator, brake line and carburetor. It's a whole other concept to know that these parts do different things to make the car run.

Sure, understanding the manner in which testosterone operates might not seem that important to you now, but just because you know that a car is a way to get from point A to point B doesn't stop you from popping the hood once in a while to take a peek. As they say, knowing is half the battle, and in the battle against the Beer Belly Blues you can use every ally you can get. If nothing else, you can save this information for unique conversational material in an absolute emergency. You may even be able to educate your health professional!

Testosterone is a lot like alcohol, and not only because we all have days where we wish there were more of it in us. While the concept of "having a drink" is fairly universal, the experience of actually doing it varies according to the delivery method employed. No one in his right mind would walk into a pub and ask the barkeep for "a cocktail" without further specification, as this could mean a whisky sour just as easily as it could mean something served in half a coconut with two-thirds of the produce section skewered on the straw. A shot of hard liquor might have the same alcohol content as a glass of wine or a bottle of beer, but they are hardly interchangeable. Similarly, although the effect of testosterone remains constant, there are variations depending on the way in which it is delivered. And these variations – as you are about to discover – can make all the difference in testosterone's impact on your physiology.

Testosterone – All Tied Up

Testosterone is a fat-soluble steroid hormone that is synthesized from cholesterol, which is why it (along with estrogen) needs to be transported around the bloodstream on special carrier proteins, one of which is called sex hormone binding globulin (SHBG). Unfortunately, once testosterone is bound to SHBG, it is unable to exert its appropriate responses upon the body (one word: erections). And the kicker is SHBG levels increase with age, and with the more fat we accumulate – especially in the belly. So higher levels are, in effect, a byproduct of the Beer Belly Blues itself. So if you were looking for a reason your erection isn't what it used to be, there you go – it's an SHBG thing, among other things.

SHBG is a plasma glycoprotein that provides the strongest bond to testosterone as it transports it throughout the bloodstream. Predominately produced by the liver (and to a much lesser extent the testes and brain), levels of SHBG are influenced by the health of the organ. This means that it can be affected by some of the same conditions we discussed earlier. Perhaps due to its comparable prevalence within the system, it comes as little surprise that researchers have singled out SHBG for further study in regard to its possible usefulness in assessing health risks associated with the Beer Belly Blues.

Because the vital role SHBG levels play when it comes to your sex-hormone status, along with the proper reading of hormone panels, it becomes increasingly important to assess SHBG levels accurately as we age. Unfortunately very few doctors understand the importance of SHBG when it comes to healthy hormone levels. therefore, even fewer of them test for its levels. No worries, I've included the latest research into what constitutes an optimal SHBG level in Part III.

Aside from its role as a master regulator of sex-hormone status, newer research is indicating that SHBG itself my act a lot like a hormone or messenger molecule in its own right. A newer study in the journal *Hormone Metabolism Research*, found that healthy SHBG levels help to increase communication between cells, and that unhealthy levels are associated with prostate disease and cancer, breast cancer, obesity, lower HDL cholesterol levels, Alzheimer's disease, osteoporosis and cardiovascular disease.

You are already very acquainted with the fact that as a man ages his testosterone levels start to diminish. What you may not be so familiar with is that as this precipitous decline is occurring and belly fat is increasing, levels of SHBG are also increasing – often right alongside the growing beer belly. This erodes testosterone levels as they become more and more stuck to the SHBG molecule. As SHBG levels increase, the activity or bioavailability of testosterone becomes further reduced, which is a major reason why total testosterone doesn't mean nearly as much as how much of that testosterone is unbound or freed from SHBG. In other words, you may still be walking around with the total testosterone levels of a twenty year old, but since the majority of that testosterone is unavailable to your tissues you'll never be the wiser for it, and obviously neither will your wilting body.

Even though heaps of research show that most men experience elevated SHBG levels with age, it is equally important not to experience SHBG levels that are too low. For instance, after reviewing decades of research German researchers showed that low SHBG levels are a predictable indicator of the metabolic syndrome, which is hallmarked by abdominal obesity, high heart disease risk and out-of-control blood sugar levels. A study appearing in the European *Journal of Endocrinology* showed that both low total testosterone and low SHBG are strong predictors of the metabolic syndrome in men. According to researchers from the National Public Health Institute in Finland, the problem becomes exacerbated when you consider studies that show a direct link between increased insulin levels and lowered SHBG status, as increased insulin is almost always associated with metabolic syndrome.

Get Your Coffee Fix?

UCLA researchers recently evaluated the purported link between drinking coffee and a reduced risk of diabetes. Aside from the research-proven blood-sugar lowering effects of chlorogenic acid in coffee, it was discovered that coffee stimulated the production of SHBG, something scientists believed to be directly related to the fact that subjects who consumed four or more cups of coffee a day developed diabetes at a rate less than half of that reflected by their non-coffee-drinking counterparts. According to one of the lead researchers, "We now know that this protein, SHBG, is critical as an early target for assessing the risk and prevention of the onset of diabetes ... the lower the levels of SHBG, the greater the risk beyond any known diabetes risk factors." It has also been identified as a means by which one might predict the likelihood of bone fractures, particularly in men suffering from osteoporosis.

Furthermore, SHBG is the form of testosterone used in the equation to calculate one's Free Androgen Index (FAI), a measure of the normalcy of one's sex hormone levels. In the irrefutably scientific terminology of the Three Stooges, this would make SHBG the Larry of the testosterone-form stooges.

Albumin – The Not-So-Bad Testosterone Transporter

Albumin, also referred to as serum albumin by those who are paid by the letter, is the most common form of blood protein found in the human body. In addition to testosterone, it carries in its many arms numerous other molecules, such as fatty acids and even medicines, while loudly singing the theme from *The Bodyguard*. Though it doesn't receive the same attention as its showboating cohort SHBG, albumin is still regarded as having a considerable amount of statistical importance unto itself. Its levels have been specifically accounted for in research concerning erectile dysfunction, and its levels are a strong indicator of both overall health and mortality. Numerous studies indicate that both the levels of albumin-bound testosterone and free (biologically active) testosterone – the most powerful form of testosterone – are the main determining factors behind testosterone bioavailability (the testosterone that makes the difference to your manliness).

And Now for the Star

Unlike SHBG and albumin-bound testosterone, free and biologically active testosterone is its own man. Still full of potential and having yet to be bound to any old nagging protein, it treats the blood stream as its very own bachelor pad, putting its feet up on the coffee table and leaving its dirty laundry laying about wherever it sees fit. Keeping in theme with its bachelorhood, the hallmark of free and biologically active testosterone is this sense of liberty. Researchers have determined that testosterone is a more reliable diagnostic indicator of overall health prior to bonding either with SHBG or serum albumin, due to the fact that it exists in its original pure state and bears none of the characteristics that come after bonding with a specialized protein.

However, its rareness greatly complicates things. While, as we now know, levels of testosterone decrease over the years, only a fraction of a percent of the remaining amount present in the male circulatory system is free and biologically active (between 0.5-3 percent). Researchers are forced to choose between the accuracy of their methodology and the cost and availability of their procedures. In response to this, scientists in Europe and Australia recently conducted studies designed to test the efficacy of alternative methods to account for free testosterone within the system, including the FAI mentioned above. Their results provided equations that produce a more accurate model of a subject's free testosterone level, ensuring an improvement in the quality and accuracy of future research. So, to sum things up as this pertains to you avoiding the Beer Belly Blues, it is always best to be footloose and fancy FREE – well, at least where your testosterone status is concerned. Along with assessing your optimal SHBG levels in Part III, I'll also provide optimal levels and testing procedures for your Total Testosterone (the measurement of all the free testosterone, albumin-bound testosterone and SHBG-bound testosterone in a given blood sample) and free-testosterone on its own.

Chapter Twelve:

Estradiol – What You Need to Know

In my award-winning book, *Beer Belly Blues*, I wrote a chapter called, Dude Looks Like a Lady, which is a takeoff from a title of a song performed by an aged rocker that, well … kinda looked like a lady! The point is, in that short chapter I brought to light a condition that is, unfortunately, the scourge of countless men who experience the Beer Belly Blues. I'm talking about the dreaded "Man Boob Syndrome," or its more technical name, *gynecomastia* – which quite literally means "woman's breast" from the Greek root words that comprise it.

Gynecomastia is actually the development of fatty breast tissue in men, and is more often than not a byproduct of low testosterone and high levels of the so-called female hormone estrogen. The condition can also be found in pre-pubescent or early-pubescent teens who find themselves with higher-than-normal estrogen levels due to excess abdominal fat. The good news is that for the majority of the younger dudes, the condition corrects itself as the boy loses body fat and becomes a man over time, but not so much in the case of middle-aged men who suddenly find themselves looking through the brassiere section of the latest edition of the Victoria's Secret catalog – and not because of the hot looking women on the pages!

So as you can see, along with the Beer Belly Blues comes a lessening of the man you once were (physiologically speaking) with an ever-increasing femininity. Lowered testosterone and heightened estrogen levels equate to a condition known as estrogen dominance. Higher levels of estrogen contribute to greater manifestation of classically feminine physical characteristics (aka Man Boobs and the inclination to power shop).

Now that you are a little more acquainted with your feminine side, let's delve a little deeper into the role estrogens play over time in your physiology and biochemistry. Estrogen is the sex hormone most prominent in females. Most women have up to forty times more of it in their bodies than men. It is the yin to testosterone's yang. "Well, that's all well and good," you might be thinking to yourself. "I've got enough on my plate as it is. Why do I need to concern myself with problems exclusive to the fairer sex?" Well, here's the deal: Estrogen is very much your problem, too, and as seems to be a recurring theme in the Beer Belly Blues, it is only worsening with age.

Relax, there's no need to panic just yet. It does not mean that you will need to start matching your shoes to your tool belt or to your brand-new purse, or TiVo'ing the upcoming Lifetime *Movie of the Week*. You are not required to forget how to parallel park your car, nor will you be expected to pluck, wax or otherwise groom an additional square inch of your body (above and beyond what you've got going on right now, that is). Just as women need some testosterone in their system as means of bolstering sexual desire – actually, testosterone is also referred to as the hormone of desire in both sexes – men naturally manufacture a small amount of estrogen within theirs. In fact, estrogen performs an important function in the male reproductive system by regulating sperm count and moderating the libido.

Aromatase – the Estrogen Manufacturer

However, that is not to say that everything is guaranteed to be perfect – in fact, far from it. As the body's chemistry begins to change, certain cellular processes begin to change along with it and, in the process, threaten to throw the system out of whack. The effects on a man's system can be quite unpleasant when experiencing *hyperestrogenemia* (estrogen dominance), both the technical term for an excessive amount of estrogen and an impressive way to win a game of Scrabble. Aside from the Man Boob Syndrome, other effects of estrogen dominance include obesity and lowered sperm counts. While an overabundance of estrogen can result from certain conditions such as Klinefelter syndrome, wherein a male possesses an extra X chromosome in addition to his standard XY pairing, it is more likely due to a pesky biochemical called aromatase.

Though it might sound like a word used by persnickety food critics in describing the combined smell and flavor of their dish, aromatase is actually the name of an enzyme that exists in various tissues of the boy such as bone, skin, brain and especially belly fat – primarily the subcutaneous layer just underneath the skin. Found both in males and females, aromatase is responsible for the creation of hormones via a process that could be arguably the grandest Benedict Arnold-ing occurring on the cellular level. It actually converts androgens (remember the mega star of the androgen world is none other than – you guessed it – testosterone) into estrogen, thus striking a double whammy against the body's efforts to maintain a gender-appropriate balance of sex hormones.

With testosterone already in short supply thanks to the Beer Belly Blues cycle, one can hardly afford to part with any unless absolutely necessary, much less transform it into its polar opposite. This effectively doubles the loss, much like being fined a buck for burning a dollar bill, tipping the scale even further away from the natural balance. Over time this adds up, and statistics have shows that men of retirement age can often have more estrogen in their bodies than women of the same age – yikes!

Sweet 16 – Only There's Nothing Sweet About It!

Decreased testosterone, elevated SHBG and increased estrogen levels are bad enough, but when you consider the fact that men also experience an increase in a very harmful form of estrogen with increased age and body fat levels (known as *16-alpha hydroxy estrone*), which increases the risk of prostate cancer and makes it extremely difficult to maintain a healthy metabolism, you quickly understand that most men need as much help as they can get in order to make it through the Beer Belly Blues.

The form of estrogen most commonly found in males, *estradiol* – and the one from which all other estrogens are manufactured – affects a wide range of features. Apart from the aforementioned reproductive system, it also has a hand in blood flow, bone formation, and even brain function. It also happens to be the type of estrogen that stimulates the development of secondary sexual characteristics in women; that is to say, those traits that, although not an active part of the reproductive system, are considered gender-specific. Think about the buck's antlers, or the lion's mane – recognizable traits that, in addition to any pragmatic purpose, serve as a readily apparent means of identifying them to other members of the species as a member of one sex or the other. As you might imagine, this effect might be viewed in a less-than-favorable light by men who find themselves perfectly content with the bosom they already have. The Beer Belly Blues are a tough enough tune to carry without the complication of trying to teach yourself how to properly put on a brassiere this late in life.

High estrogen levels in men make it harder and harder to lose excess belly fat, which further exacerbates the conditions associated with the Beer Belly Blues. And if that wasn't bad enough, high estrogen levels are also associated with a much greater risk of heart disease and early death. In fact, according to a 2010 study that appeared in the prestigious *Journal of the American Medical Association* (JAMA), men with high levels of estrogen experienced a 133-percent greater risk of death. The interesting thing about this study is it also pointed out the importance of balanced estrogen levels in men, as researchers showed that men who experienced excessively *low* estrogen levels were 317-percent more likely to die. This is yet one more reason to ensure that your hormone levels are optimal, as opposed to either too high or too low (as in the case of testosterone). I will share with you optimal estrogen (estradiol) values in Part III.

Understanding Aromatase

Researchers in New York recently undertook a study to investigate how they might halt or otherwise slow an unwanted proliferation of aromatase by examining a specific form of cancer directly related to the presence of estrogen. As aromatase is responsible for the conversion of testosterone into estrogen, they theorized that inhibiting its production would constitute a formidable preventative measure. Unfortunately, the exact molecular structure of that particular enzyme was still not fully understood, which prevented a thorough analysis of the exact process by which the cells could be manipulated. Undeterred, the researchers became the first team to crystallize aromatase, a process that provided them with the first fully-mapped atomic model of it. This allowed them a better understanding of its exact cellular structure, which gave insight into how to stop its action. They concluded that further research into the field of aromatase inhibitors would be greatly aided (by these discoveries). Too bad they didn't know about a 100-percent natural compound – which I'll discuss a bit later – that is very effective at inhibiting excess aromatase activity.

Good thing, too, because the last thing we need at this point is to start developing female features. Otherwise, between that and what we learned before, it would seem that we were running the risk of turning into the fat lady singing the Beer Belly Blues. And we just can't have that, because we aren't done yet!

Chapter Thirteen:
Cholesterol – Testosterone Fuel

As we have seen in the previous chapters, sometimes the Beer Belly Blues reads like a sheet of classical music. Cluttered with foreign words and abbreviations such as hypogonadism and SHBG, some of the material covered might seem better suited to the maestros of biology to whom these concepts are no more daunting than a simple A. Rather than doing our part in contributing to the betterment of our lives, this sense of defeatism provides a handy excuse for succumbing to the myriad effects of testosterone loss including, as we discussed in chapter 7, the tendency to "B-flat," both musically and otherwise. However, rather than just sitting around and scratching our piccolos in utter confusion, we can use the information to take charge of our situation and our health.

Other times we are more fortunate, and the Beer Belly Blues sound a little closer to "Mary Had A Little Lamb" – being old makes us tired, exercising builds muscle, and our hair looks better on the top of our heads than it does circling around the bottom of our drains. Another one of these – if television commercials are to be trusted (and how could they not?!) – would be that cholesterol is evil and to be exterminated with extreme prejudice. After all, we are fully commited ton the "so-called" fact that it's stuffing up our veins, clogging up our hearts, and cutting down our lifespan. Heck, why stop there? Might as well blame all those missing socks and car keys on cholesterol while we're at it. In short, cholesterol is all evil and should be stopped at all costs. But what if we are wrong about cholesterol – what if we are dead wrong?!

What is Cholesterol?

If you can think back to the '80s, you might remember a very strange period in which eggs went from being great for you to being awful for you, and then back again. The reason behind this is the cholesterol component of the egg yolk, or more specifically, the misunderstanding of it.

At the chemical level, cholesterol is classified as a steroid, just like testosterone, and is a member of a subgroup known as the *sterol* alcohols.

It is a waxy organic substance, which happens to be a major component of cell membranes in all animal tissues (yes, including us), which is why the body deems it important enough to manufacture so much of the stuff (close to 1,000 milligrams every day, or the equivalent of four to five eggs). Cholesterol derivatives (phytosterols) are important to certain plants and fungi, and are essential in a number of cellular functions. Cholesterol is necessary for constructing and repairing the membranes that protect the inner processes of the cells, as well as facilitating these processes via providing transportation throughout the cell and assisting in cellular communication.

Additionally, cholesterol is a vital element in the production of vitamin D and bile. It also happens to be the major building block of sex hormones such as – you guessed it – testosterone.

After all the time we have spent singing the praises of testosterone (hey, we needed a break from the Beer Belly Blues), you might guess that this is the point at which I explain why cholesterol isn't all that evil. I mean, it's obviously in charge of some very important things, so how in the world could it have possibly gotten such a bad rap?

Forms of Cholesterol

Part of the problem stems from those who have only a partial understanding of cholesterol and how it works. Cholesterol (again, like testosterone) comes in several different forms, each of which performs a unique function and behaves differently within the body. These forms, in turn, are designated in terms of their lipoprotein structure. Lipoproteins, which consist of a combination of lipids (or fat molecules) and proteins (err, self-explanatory), exist in the following five forms:

Chylomicrons, the largest of the lipoproteins, are produced in the small intestine and carry *exogenous* lipids (those derived from the diet as opposed to manufactured internally) to your muscles, heart and liver.

Very low-density Lipoprotein (VLDL), which transports endogenous lipids (those derived from the body) throughout the body. VLDLs are larger and filled with triglycerides (which we will discuss momentarily), and eventually degrade into IDLs.

Intermediate Density Lipoprotein (IDL) is formed after VLDLs depart with the majority of their triglycerides. If not recycled to the liver, IDLs proceed through the bloodstream and become LDLs.

Low Density Lipoprotein (LDL), or as it is more commonly known, "bad cholesterol," is the poster child for prejudice against cholesterol, as it is frequently associated with the heightened risk of heart disease and other similar health problems. There are actually two forms of LDL, known as types A and B, the latter of which is considered somewhat more dangerous.

High Density Lipoprotein (HDL), the white knight of the blood stream.

Now that we know not all cholesterol is bad, let's discuss how we can separate what is from what isn't.

HDL vs. LDL

When asked about the risks of cholesterol, the most frequent response is that it can clog up the arteries. In fact, it is the LDL which tends to do the clogging, whereas the smaller HDL assists in its removal – much like a tiny piece of floss is able to slip in between teeth and dislodge a larger chunk of food. This sort of "Goofus and Gallant"-type binary remains consistent across the board. Whereas the absorption of LDL particles into the walls of arteries leads to the plaque build-up that can result in a stroke or heart attack, the Framingham Heart Study – one of the longest ongoing cardiovascular studies that began in 1948 – concluded that patients testing for high levels of cholesterol within their HDL particles, or HDL-C, showed a reduced risk of death.

Due to the considerable difference between the LDL and HDL, it should come as little surprise that one's total combined level of cholesterol is nowhere near as important to understanding the implications on one's health as is the ratio of HDL to LDL. In a healthy adult male, at least 40 milligrams of HDL-C per 1 deciliter of blood is considered good. From this level, assuming you possess the ideal level of LDL-C dictated by the Framingham Heart Study, (100 mg/dL), every additional milligram of HDL-C added per milligram of blood reduces the risk of heart disease by up to 3 percent. This ratio remains consistent both in the positive and negative sense, with lower ratios of HDL to LDL leading to a heightened risk.

Antioxidant support is also a crucial consideration in monitoring a healthy level of cholesterol, as some studies show that LDL must first be altered or oxidized before it becomes problematic. One example of oxidized LDL particles is when you fry or scramble eggs at high temperatures versus poaching or boiling them, which greatly limits the damage to the cholesterol component. Specialized enzymes found in fruits and vegetables have been shown to protect existing levels of LDL and

HDL from further damage or depletion, not to mention hints of greater potential use. For instance, researchers recently investigated potential ties between antioxidant usage in conjunction with cholesterol therapy for patients suffering from certain cardiovascular afflictions and the consensus is that antioxidants may impact heart health in a very positive manner.

The Real Culprit

So if it truly isn't the cholesterol level to blame for our heart disease and unpaid parking tickets, then what is it? Carbohydrates and triglycerides are two likely suspects.

A quick stroll through the diet section of your local bookstore would lead you to believe that carbohydrates are the worst thing for your diet since butter-fried bacon brownies (I haven't performed a Google search on these. However I am pretty sure they exist somewhere in North America). As we learned above, it just isn't that simple, and the right kinds of carbohydrates do, in fact, play a meaningful role in the proper function of your anatomy.

According to the World Health Organization (WHO) and the Food and Agriculture Organization, 55-75 percent of an adult's daily caloric intake should come from carbohydrates such as those contained in bread, pasta, beans and rice. While this might seem all well and good, carbohydrates may pose more of a problem when it comes to exacerbating the Beer Belly Blues. Carbohydrates, while convenient, may not necessarily be needed for the body to function – which is why there is no recommended daily allowance (RDA) for carbohydrates in our diet. Our bodies can derive all their energy from fat and protein, which are both also necessary for construction on a molecular level (unlike carbohydrates). Aside from this fact, carbohydrates like the ones mentioned above provide a high-glycemic load to the diet, ultimately leading to high circulating levels of blood sugar (think pre-diabetes) and excess body fat in the – you guessed it again – beer-belly region.

The Glycemic Load or Index?

Numerous health professionals still use the outdated Glycemic Index to establish whether an individual carbohydrate is going to spike blood sugar levels or not. However, newer research shows that the Glycemic Load is a much better indicator of how these foods affect blood sugar and insulin. The Glycemic Load of a food is calculated by multiplying the glycemic index by a 100-gram serving of the carbohydrate in question. Prior to the glycemic load, foods that had a reading of over 70 were avoided like the plague, whereas their glycemic load readings didn't show nearly the same degree of potential problems.

What carbohydrates do contribute is a readily-available form of energy that can be burned in the place of protein or fat. Unfortunately, this means that when consumed in excess or in the wrong forms (i.e. high glycemic loads), carbohydrates can supplant the amount of fat that would regularly be burned, leading it instead to be stored away for later use usually as body fat. As you might imagine, this can lead to all sorts of difficulty, ranging from a second Battle of the Bulge (excess carbohydrates can easily be converted into the most prevalent form of fat in the body – triglycerides) to *hypercholesterolemia*, a disorder caused when carbohydrates that are unable to be effectively burned or stored trigger high blood sugar levels, the storage of extra body fat (a condition closely associated with high insulin and blood sugar levels), or even a heart attack.

You can easily control blood sugar levels by remaining conscious of your intake of carbohydrates – particularly in limiting your intake of simple and overly refined carbohydrates such as those found in soft drinks, candy, potato chips, white flour and cornmeal-based products – and favoring fresh, fibrous vegetables and fruits (primarily from the berry family, due to their low glycemic load) as your primary choice. In the process you can lower excess insulin, LDL cholesterol and start reducing that keg around your waist.

Whole Grains – Not So Fast!

Grains – especially the so-called nutritious ones such as whole grains – have been recommended by dietitians and other health experts since we can all last remember. One primary reason for this is because respected governmental organizations like The United States Department of Agriculture (USDA) recommends that we consume copious amounts of these grains, and health professionals blindly trust in these recommendations – often without looking at the research. For instance, the USDA recommends a daily consumption of 8 ounces of daily grains for men and 6 ounces for women. Unfortunately, almost all grains stimulate too much insulin and blood sugar, which makes them bad choices when getting rid of the beer belly. Aside from this, newer research is showing that wheat and other grains are not nearly as nutritious as we've been led to believe and that they may actually be hazardous to our health.

Triglycerides, on the other hand, are fatty chemical compounds found predominately in animal fats and vegetable oils. They are used primarily to store calories that have otherwise gone unused, such as those found in proteins left over from a diet high in carbohydrates (which is, in fact, one of the conditions most closely associated with high triglyceride counts). Triglycerides, as mentioned above, are also a main component of body fat and VLDLs, and therefore contribute to the production of extra LDL within the system, compromising the almighty HDL-LDL ratio. Having an excess in triglycerides can lead to *hypertriglyceridemia*, a condition related to both pancreatitis and atherosclerosis. Minor lifestyle changes, such as limiting the intake of alcohol and excess carbohydrates while supplementing your diet with omega-3 fatty acids (such as those found in hempseed, flaxseed and primarily molecularly distilled fish oils), can be made to keep triglycerides in check.

The absolute importance of maintaining a proper cholesterol ratio can be especially troubling to those having difficulty preserving a healthy level of testosterone, as numerous studies have shown HDL levels to be directly correlated to those of testosterone. In addition, low levels of testosterone have been shown to impair the efficiency of the liver in filtering excessive amounts of cholesterol from the bloodstream, as well as hindering HDL in reducing the arterial build-up of LDL. A Turkish study published in the 2007 issue of the *Journal of Coronary Artery Disease* also linked low levels of free testosterone with the development of early onset heart disease. Conversely, The Rotterdam Study showed that in a group of 504 men ranging in age from 67 to 75, those experiencing the lowest rate of coronary artery disease were one in the same as those with the highest levels of free bio-available testosterone.

If, for some reason, you still aren't sold on the premise of cholesterol as a good guy, let's take a look at what happens when we go overboard in our quest to regulate it.

Chapter Fourteen:
The Truth about Statins

Though the practice of using snake oil for medicinal purposes might date back as far as Ancient Egypt, the concept of the snake-oil salesman is perhaps most closely identified with the traveling hucksters that preyed upon the naiveté of American pioneers. During the building of the American Transcontinental railroad, Chinese laborers were known to treat joint pain with … well, snake oil, a practice they passed along to their European counterparts. Noting the growing popularity of the remedy, certain less-scrupulous individuals built entire business empires on their personal "re-creations" of the alleged cure-all, most of which carried absolutely no medicinal benefit beyond the possible placebo effect. Hmmm, kinda reminds me of the pharmaceutical industry. A pervasive element of the social consciousness of the times, snake oil pops up quite memorably in Mark Twain's *Adventures of Tom Sawyer*, wherein once a day Aunt Polly forces Tom to take a "pain killer," as it will do him well. He is excused from doing so, however, upon feeding his daily dose to the cat, causing it to behave bizarrely.

Up until the 1906 Food and Drugs Act, there remained little recourse against these shysters. Few controls existed to regulate them and the sale of their useless medicines. Outside of running them out of town on a rail once their scam was uncovered, the consequences were slim to none. Due to the fact that there are modern safeguards in place – such as governmental oversight and extensive trial periods for potential medications – one would believe that we are safe from falling victim to such crude schemes as taking a medicine we don't need, and which may actually carry effects more harmful than good. However, according to a group of leading health researchers – appearing in a research paper titled "Death by Medicine," funded by the Nutrition Institute of America (a nonprofit independent research organization), nearly 800,000 Americans die each year due to side effects caused by conventional medicine. That is more than the total number of people who die in America each year from the previously believed number-one killer, heart disease (699,697 people). Now let's take a look at the widespread proliferation of the widely believed-to-be miracle drugs: statins.

What Are Statins?

Statins are a group of drugs that actually block the body's ability to manufacture cholesterol. As we discussed in the previous chapter, cholesterol has become somewhat of a bogeyman in modern health circles. Despite the obvious benefits – one of which is maintaining healthy levels of testosterone – of maintaining a healthy level of cholesterol within the bloodstream (and in particular, a healthy ratio of HDL to LDL), the relatively widespread disinformation regarding cholesterol allows it to be exploited as a scapegoat for other conditions such as obesity and cardiovascular disease. Subsequently enterprising pharmaceutical companies and doctors capitalize on it.

Statins exist in several different forms – *atorvastatin*, *fluvastatin*, *lovastatin*, *pitavastatin*, *pravastatin*, *rosuvastatin*, and *simvastatin* – and are marketed under well-known brand names such as Lescol, Lipostat, Lipitor and Crestor. As of 2003, atorvastatin became the best-selling pharmaceutical in the world. Produced by Pfizer under the names Lipitor and Torva, sales of these drugs accounted for more than $12 billion in 2008 alone.

Despite their irrefutable commercial popularity, controversy exists as to whether or not statins are worth the considerable amount of money spent on them. Though intended to be used when conventional methods such as dieting and exercise fail to provide the desired results – even though diet does not really have very much to do with the cholesterol that's produced within your body and accounts for the vast majority of the stuff – there is evidence that statins are overprescribed and end up being taken instead of pursuing natural (and side-effect-free) methods of maintaining a healthy cholesterol status. Furthermore, studies have yet to provide conclusive evidence as to their effectiveness in different scenarios.

Perhaps the most compelling argument for the use of statins can be made based on cases of patients either already diagnosed with or considered at high risk for developing cardiovascular diseases, as numerous attempts have been made to link the use of statins to a decrease in the frequency of strokes as well as that of ischemic heart disease (IHD) – events such as heart attack and heart failure. In a study performed by the University of London, the use of statins to lower LDL in 164 subjects led to a 60 percent reduction in occurrences of IHD and a 17-percent reduction in strokes.

However, investigations into the use of statins have just as frequently yielded less conclusive, or even conflicting, results. On one hand, researchers at the University of Alberta found that statins could reduce the risk of death and certain cholesterol-related diseases in patients considered to be at a "low cardiovascular risk" at the same rate as it could in patients with a history of coronary artery disease. On the other, a separate study conducted at the University of Cambridge in England found no evidence that statin therapy provided a tangible benefit for even those considered to be in high-risk scenarios.

This inconsistency could perhaps be accounted for based on the results of another recent study in England, this one by the London School of Hygiene and Tropical Medicine. While their results seemed to conclude that statins contributed to a number of factors, including an overall decrease in patient mortality, their findings may have been mitigated by procedural shortcomings such as subjects misreporting their own conditions and the inclusion of subjects with preexisting conditions. As research into this subject remains murky at best, perhaps for now it might be more advantageous to focus on what we do know about statins than what we do not.

How Statins Work

As mentioned above, statins are designed to reduce the level of cholesterol within the bloodstream. They do so by interacting with *HMG-CoA reductase*, an enzyme essential for the production of cholesterol within the liver, particularly through a process known as competitive inhibition.

Imagine the production of cholesterol in terms of a drive-through car wash on a microscopic level. The available active site on the enzyme HMG-CoA reductase is the "car wash" itself, whereas the "dirty car" is represented by the substrate molecule. In order to produce cholesterol (or a "clean car"), a dirty car must first pull in to the car wash so that it can be "cleaned" (transformed to a separate end-product via a catalytic reaction). Keeping in theme, statins work somewhat like a broken-down school bus stuck inside the car wash, or a well-placed stack of bricks. If the car wash is blocked, the dirty car cannot pull in, and therefore it cannot emerge as the sort of clean car that will lead to a later increase in testosterone levels.

By effectively blocking substrate molecules from interacting with HMG-CoA reductase enzymes, statins reduce the body's ability to manufacture cholesterol, a situation that comes with a number of risks.

Statins Are Risky Business

The correspondence between a variety of ailments and taking statins is well-documented but somewhat overlooked; in fact, a study conducted at the University of California suggested that doctors tend to under-report these side effects at a statistically significant rate, meaning they are even more prevalent than we might think.

Apart from the obvious risk of interfering with the delicate balance of the body's chemistry by introducing a foreign substance, statins are associated with a number of health issues – some of which greatly impact the Beer Belly Blues. Remember, testosterone is derived from cholesterol, and therefore any undue reduction in cholesterol can lead to the conditions specific to testosterone loss. However, it doesn't end there.

According to the Mayo Clinic, the most common side effect of taking a statin is muscle pain. Ranging from discomfort to debilitating, the pain might be described as tiredness, soreness or weakness. Rarely, and most commonly in conjunction with taking other medications, one might experience *rhabdomyolysis*, a conditioned marked by intense muscle pain, kidney failure and possibly death.

Another risk of taking statins is the potential for impairment in the function of the liver. The liver is where cholesterol is both manufactured and inhibited. The forcible alteration of its day-to-day operations can interfere with the liver's regulatory capabilities, causing it to produce additional enzymes in an attempt to compensate for what the body interprets as a chemical deficiency. Elevated enzyme counts can prove quite harmful once they reach a critical level.

According to an Italian study published in 1993, the use of statins by an individual can reduce his levels of Coenzyme Q10 (CoQ10) by up to 40 percent. CoQ10 is an important component of the electron transport chain and participates in ATP. If you can think way, way back to high school science class, you might recall this as an important process in generating energy for the human body on a cellular level, most importantly in high-demand organs such as the brain, kidney and liver. Decreases in the amount of CoQ10 lead to premature aging and energy loss and the potential for diminished function within the organs and certain systems.

Natural Alternatives to Statins

In short, avoid statins if possible. Too often these days, doctors are willing to prescribe first and ask questions later. Rather than simply accept them at face value, do not be afraid to request alternative therapies or seek them out on your own. Several natural alternatives to statins not only exist but are readily available. For instance:

- Plant sterols and stanols (beta-sitosterol) are natural cholesterol-like substances found in the plant kingdom. These plant chemicals resemble cholesterol (on a molecular level) and because of this feature, they can prevent bad cholesterol from being absorbed into your bloodstream. Numerous studies confirm the effectiveness of plant sterols and stanols in reducing cholesterol naturally. One such proven product, called Immuno-Care, has been the subject of clinical trials at the University of Guelph in Canada. Researchers found that Immuno-Care is very effective in reducing circulating levels of LDL-cholesterol and increasing circulating levels of HDL-cholesterol.

- Niacin (vitamin B3) is known to reduce the ratio of LDL to HDL within the bloodstream by preventing the breakdown of fats.

- Dietary fiber, as it is digested, yields short-chain fatty acids (SCFA), which, along with the added benefits of stabilizing blood sugar levels and stimulating the immune system, also reduces LDL. Look for 100 percent organic fiber blends.

- Citrus and palm fruit extracts have been shown to favorably impact levels of LDL, HDL and triglycerides. Look for the patented research-proven brand, Sytrinol.

If, for some reason, the use of statins is deemed absolutely necessary, it is still wise to take measures in order to counteract negative effects. CoQ10 supplements, in addition to boosting energy by restoring levels diminished by statins, have been shown to prevent heart failure, improve blood pressure, and are even being investigated as a treatment for cancer.

Fortunately it is quite easy to integrate CoQ10 into your daily diet. Supplements in the form of ubiquinol have been shown to greatly and enhance bodily CoQ10 levels. Also, organic grass-fed meats and healthy vegetable oil (think olive) are all CoQ10-rich. Frying should be avoided in their preparation, as this lowers the CoQ10 content by up to 32 percent.

So now you know the dastardly truth about statins. But you should also know that testosterone-supporting meals – from my Beer Belly Blues Diet – will help teach your body how to maintain a healthy ratio of HDL to LDL cholesterol so that you can fight off the Beer Belly Blues and say NO to statins once and for all. I'll show you how in Part III.

Chapter Fifteen:
The Truth about ED Drugs

As you get older, the odds of running into our not-so-welcome friend ED increase dramatically. According to a study published in the *Journal of Urology*, the likelihood of experiencing erectile dysfunction (either physically or in the form of reduced libido) in your 60s is as much as four times greater than it is in your 40s. With a wide range of risk factors including surgery, stress, high blood pressure and lifestyle choices (think laziness, alcohol and tobacco use), it is easy to see how those of us going through the Beer Belly Blues are all especially at danger.

Considering the extremely personal nature of the problems caused by ED, one might think that those afflicted would go out of their way to avoid professional treatment, preferring to suffer in silence rather than going through the embarrassment of dealing with their problems face to face. A 2002 article appearing in the *Wall Street Journal* indicated that 80 percent of men never seek treatment for their condition, but a lot can change in a little over a decade.

The truth of the matter seems to now be quite the opposite. As I discussed in the earlier chapter on the "unit," erectile dysfunction is now such a widespread ailment that there is very little social stigma against it; in fact, it is a well-known problem that is generally accepted as a side effect of the lowering testosterone levels that occur alongside aging.

In fact, drugs designed to treat erectile dysfunction make up a sizable proportion of the prescription medicines sold today. Part of this is inevitable, as ED afflicts a wide demographic and therefore would naturally be more popular than drugs used in the treatment of rarer conditions. Another part of this stems from the psychological aspect of ED, as many feel ashamed of what might be perceived as their inability to perform and would go to any lengths to avoid embarrassment. Still another part is just the simple fact that there's no sense in missing out on all that fun if it can be prevented by just taking a pill or two. Whatever the reason, the unfortunate truth of the situation is that despite their popularity, prescription remedies for erectile dysfunction are not all they are cracked up to be.

Cialis

Tadalafil, marketed by Eli Lilly and Company as Cialis, was approved for sale by the United States Food and Drug Administration in November of 2003, making it the newest of the three most frequently-prescribed ED drugs (the other two are mentioned below). It is known for its 36-hour window of effectiveness (as compared to the shorter effectiveness of its competitors), having been dubbed "The Weekend Pill." Cialis is noteworthy for being the only of the three main ED drugs to be recommended for use not only on an as-need basis, but also as part of a daily regimen. It is also marketed as a treatment for pulmonary arterial hypertension under the trade name Adcirca and, as of October 2011, has been approved for use in the treatment of benign prostatic hyperplasia. Kinda makes one wonder what other areas this pharmaceutical giant will try to exploit?

Cialis is perhaps most famous for being the first of the main erectile dysfunction drugs to include newly-required language mandated by the Food and Drug Administration regarding an expanded list of potential side effects, including *priapism* (an unusually long and often painful errection, leading to the condition otherwise accepted as the Awkward Boner Syndrome). Much to the chagrin of certain family organizations, some of these ads debuted during the 2004 Super Bowl; however, any potential controversy regarding such adult-oriented content being presented to an audience with a large proportion of children was overshadowed by the infamous "Wardrobe Malfunction" halftime show. It has also been a major advertiser in the world of golf, sponsoring both the PGA Tour and the America's Cup.

Side effects common to Cialis include flushing of the skin, runny or stuffy nose, indigestion, headache and back pain.

Levitra

Sold by Bayer as Levitra, vardenafil is also known as Vivanza (in Italy) and Staxyn (when presented in an orally-soluble form). In addition to erectile dysfunction, vardenafil is also used in the treatment of premature ejaculation (Didn't your mother ever teach you that it's impolite to show up to a party early?).

While most commonly associated with nausea, vardenafil has also been tied to a wide variety of unpleasant symptoms including:

- **localized pain,** especially in the abdomen, back and eyes

- **facial edema,** or swelling from the accumulation of fluid under the skin

- **vision problems,** such as sight abnormalities and photosensitivity

- **skin problems,** such as irritation, rashes, and itching

- **cardiopulmonary issues,** such as heart palpitations, irregular heartbeat, hypotension (low blood pressure), and tachycardia (racing pulse)

- In a small number of cases, vardenafil has been involved in more severe problems such as priapism (which, if left untreated, can lead to permanent impotence) and even heart attacks.

Viagra

By far the most well-known of the three major erectile dysfunction drugs, Viagra is a form of sildenafil citrate sold by U.S. pharmaceutical giant Pfizer. After being invented by British scientists and put on sale in 1998, it has gone on to dominate the ED market, accounting for over ninety percent of it by the year 2000. Though the introduction of competitors such as Cialis and Levitra has weakened its stronghold in recent years, Viagra still remains synonymous with erectile dysfunction treatment, as witnessed by the number of knockoffs and imitators available both on the black market and over the counter, presented as herbal remedies (through frequently adulterated with synthesized materials that act in the same manner as their prescription counterparts).

Viagra has been successfully used to treat those suffering from ED due to other causes such as depression and diabetes. Outside of the realm of sexual dysfunction, it has also been prescribed for pulmonary arterial hypertension, a rare cardiac disease, and high-altitude pulmonary edema, a symptom of altitude sickness experienced most frequently by mountain climbers. It has also been researched as a cure for jet lag (of course it has).

Side effects of Viagra include a wide range of vision problems, specifically impairment, blurriness, photophobia, and the infamous "blue vision" (cyanopsia), wherein everything in one's field of vision becomes tilted a shade reminiscent of the iconic diamond-shaped pill. Other symptoms include flushed skin, indigestion and headache. Also, you might want to know that testosterone loss makes it very difficult for drugs like Viagra to work effectively, as the blood cannot be trapped in the penile arteries without testosterone

Beyond its appropriate use, Viagra has found popularity on the party circuit, being taken by those with no medical need to do so (mostly teenagers). Its reputation leads to its use in order to counteract the side effects of recreational drugs such as MDMA, ecstasy and alcohol, all of which can lead to temporary erectile dysfunction. While it has not been clinically proven to have any profoundly beneficial effect for those not suffering from chronic ED, it does provide the opportunity for danger. When taken in conjunction with certain drugs, such as "poppers" (amyl nitrites), the chemical reaction between the two can prove fatal.

Why Natural Alternatives Are Better

Besides the problems listed above, there are a few other reasons that ED prescription medications can hardly be considered a cure-all for the problems brought on by the Beer Belly Blues. As all three fall under the category of PDE5 (*phosphodiesterase* type 5) inhibitors, the USDA has linked them to both non-arthritic anterior ischemic optic neuropathy, a condition which impairs blood flow to the optic nerve and can lead to permanent damage, and an increased risk of sudden hearing loss. Complications can also arise when used in conjunction with certain other medications (especially blood thinners, nitrates and nitrites) by those who have recently experienced a stroke or heart attack, or by individuals with other impairments of the heart or liver.

Furthermore, those suffering from severe testosterone deficiencies due to the Beer Belly Blues might not get any use out of the medications, as a baseline level of testosterone is prerequisite to their function. At best you will be fleeced out of a few bucks and left in the same unfortunate condition as before; at worst, you will unnecessarily expose yourself to wide variety of health risks and potential complications, some of which are quite dangerous, or even deadly.

Fortunately there is a simple way to avoid all the problems that come along with these prescription medications: DON'T TAKE THEM. Sure, they are heavily advertised and frequently suggested by doctors, but keep in mind whom stands to profit from this: pretty much everyone but you. Rather than endanger your own well-being by succumbing to commercial pressure, why not take a moment to consider the alternatives, specifically the natural ones? I'll be discussing those next.

Chapter Sixteen:

//////////////// **Testosterone-Enhancing Nutrition – Fat Fuel**

No matter how well-designed or properly-maintained it might be, a machine is only as good as the fuel that's powering it. After all, you wouldn't expect to hit Mach-2 in an F-16 with a tank full of 87 unleaded, would you? The same goes for the human body. During a period as trying as the Beer Belly Blues, you're going to need to do a little better than pork rinds and milkshakes if you hope to achieve and maintain your ideal health status. While this may not sound ideal, a simple explanation of the basic biochemistry that defines a proper diet might help to explain why what you eat (or do not eat) is of the utmost importance.

A great number of the body's internal processes are affected by input from external sources, as anyone who has ever put down a plate of cheese fries and a case of lager in an evening will be more than happy to tell you. For instance, three-quarters of the body's total cholesterol is manufactured in the liver, leaving the rest to be obtained through one's dietary choices. If these are not carefully monitored, it can lead either to a deficit in the amount of total cholesterol (in turn leaving a shortage of material that is able to be turned into testosterone) or an abundance of it (which can lead to the storage of excessive fat, affecting internal organs such as the liver and compromising its ability to perform core functions, such as manufacturing testosterone). To put it lightly, the balance is a delicate one.

Fortunately, armed with the proper knowledge and a little bit of planning, it is entirely possible to develop a properly balanced diet that satisfies not only your basic health needs but also ensures the best chance to maintain or even enhance your testosterone levels. The best place to start this program is at the ground floor of nutrition, specifically one of the two building blocks that make up nearly everything we eat: fat.

What is Fat?

When we hear "fat," it is easy for the mind to immediately translate that as adipose tissue, or that stuff we seem to have trouble hiding under our T-shirts now that they all suddenly feel so small. Almost universally regarded as a dirty word in terms of dieting, fat actually plays an important role in a number of our important biological systems. Without it, we would be unable to derive nutrients from Vitamins A, D, E or K. The essential fatty acids – omega-3 and omega-6, a key part of one's daily nutritional requirement – are impossible for the human body to synthesize and must be consumed as part of one's dietary regimen. Fat also helps promote the health of hair and skin, can aid in protecting against disease by acting as a jail for harmful organisms, and even serves as padding and insulation, protecting the organs from trauma while helping to keep a proper temperature. In short, fat is a lot more than what's keeping you out of that old pair of jeans stuffed in the back of your closet.

However, that is not to say that all fat is a good thing all the time (i.e. the beer belly). Let's look at a few different types of fats as well as their functions within the human body.

Unsaturated vs. Saturated Fats

All dietary fats are triglycerides (remember those?) formed from fatty acids and glycerol, they can be divided into one of two categories, either *unsaturated* or *saturated*. If you're anything like the majority of North Americans, the thought of "saturated fat" conjures up images of late-night pizza boxes soaked through with grease and regret. Obviously saturated fat has to be bad, right?

Well, not exactly. The real difference between unsaturated and saturated fats is a matter of atomic construction, with saturation not referring to state of greasiness so much as how the fat molecule is arranged. As you might imagine, this is a somewhat difficult distinction to make with the naked eye. Luckily it is not the only difference between the two.

Any Vacancies?

In saturated fat, the carbon atoms making up the fat molecule are bonded to as many of its counterpart hydrogen atoms as possible (meaning there is no more space left – as in the molecule is saturated), whereas the carbon chains constituting unsaturated fats are characterized by double bonds (meaning there is one or more vacancies on the molecule).

Unsaturated Fats

For those who don't know any better, unsaturated fats are generally considered the healthier of the two forms. In fact, a 2005 study concluded that unsaturated fats, particularly those found in sunflower oil and olive oil, were an important factor in cholesterol-lowering diets. We can further subdivide unsaturated fats into two more categories: *monounsaturated* and *polyunsaturated*.

Mono-Unsaturated Fats

The lonelier-sounding of the unsaturated fats, mono-unsaturated fats are commonly found in red meat, dairy products, nuts, and more-fatty fruits such as avocados and olives. Oils are also an excellent source of monounsaturated fats, especially olive, canola, sesame and peanut oil.

Mono-unsaturated fats, when consumed in the proper ratio, have been shown to promote testosterone by decreasing LDL in relation to HDL. The aforementioned study, performed at Messiah College in Pennsylvania, showed that a diet high in monounsaturated fats could lead to a decrease in LDL by as much as 5.8 percent over the course of four weeks.

Polyunsaturated Fats

While the name might lead you to believe they can be found in crackers (yes, that was a bird joke; and no, I am not apologizing for it), polyunsaturated fats are most commonly found in nuts (such as walnuts and peanuts), seeds (sunflower or sesame), leafy greens, olive oil, fish and seaweed.

Though fine in moderation, polyunsaturated fats tend to decrease testosterone levels when consumed in excess. Additionally, polyunsaturated fats have been tied to an increased risk of certain forms of cancer.

Saturated Fats

There are four main types of dietary saturated fats:

- **Myristic Acid** - Found in nutmeg, vegetable oils and butter fats, as well as in trace amounts in a variety of animal fats.

- **Palmitic Acid** - Found in palm trees and their products (palm kernel oil, coconut oil). Primarily used as an inexpensive ingredient in soaps and cosmetics, but also as an additive in organic products and, interestingly enough, a key ingredient in napalm (hence the -palm to the na- of naphtheate).

- **Stearic Acid** - Found predominately in animal fats, but also cocoa butter and shea butter. A 2010 University of Cincinnati study suggested a link between it and low LDL levels.

- **Lauric Acid** - Most commonly found in vegetable oils such as coconut, laurel and palm kernel, though also in smaller amounts in cow and goat milk. Shown to boost HDL levels, making it a fat preferable even to unsaturated forms.

Apart from the individual benefits offered by the latter two forms, these fats, when consumed at a healthy ratio (no more than 15 percent of one's daily calories) are known to contribute to the maintenance of one's testosterone level. Main sources of saturated fat include animal products (such as meat, butter and eggs), chocolate and nuts.

Innocent Until Proven Guilty

Probably no thanks to misconceptions like my pizza example above, saturated fats tend to be regarded as the worse form of fat. However, they are not as big a risk factor as the public is led to believe. While not to be avoided entirely, the general consensus is that saturated fats should be consumed in moderation. The World Health Organization (WHO) and the governmental "so-called" nutritional gurus recommend that no more than 10 percent of one's daily caloric intake should come from saturated fats, whereas the American Health Association sets that figure somewhat lower, at 7 percent. Unfortunately, this comes into conflict with our very heredity, as the prehistoric hunting-and-gathering ancestors from whom we derive our physiology and biochemistry set the precedent for saturated fat intake at a figure closer to 15.1 percent of one's total daily allowance. Judging from the benefits listed above, is it possible that our distant relatives knew something intuitively that modern scientists tend to ignore?

Trans Fats – Testosterone Robbers

The real danger in fats, it seems, comes not from the saturated fats so much as a form of unsaturated fat known as trans fats or, as I like to call them, FrankenFats (because they are man-made atrocities). While their unique chemical structure is rare in nature, they are most likely to result from steps taken in the production of artificial foodstuffs. The main culprits, such as fast food and snack food, tend to contain high levels of trans fats due to the process of *hydrogenation*, wherein unsaturated fats such as those found in vegetable oils are chemically altered to become saturated fats. While this makes these partially hydrogenated items less prone to spoilage and suitable for storage under less-exacting climate conditions, it also makes them far more dangerous to consume.

The New England Journal of Health published a study in 2006 that asserted trans fats were more likely to elevate the risk of coronary heart disease than any other macronutrient common to the human diet. Trans fats not only elevate levels of LDL but also decrease HDL, a problem I addressed in the previous chapter on cholesterol. Studies have also shown trans fats to have a deleterious effect on the liver function, which would further impair the body's ability to produce testosterone. Other problems thought to be attributable to the excessive consumption of trans fats include depression, obesity, diabetes and cancer (hmmm, sounds like another laundry list for the Beer Belly Blues).

Fortunately the risks of trans fats are becoming more and more a matter of public knowledge, and an increasing number of manufacturers are insisting on replacing them with safer alternatives. While they might never be eliminated altogether, sticking to a diet composed predominately of natural foods will help you avoid exposing yourself to their dangerous effects.

Coconut Oil

A long-time staple of world cuisine because of its widespread availability, coconut oil has been described by food experts as "even milder and richer tasting than butter, sweeter and lighter textured than lard, and without any of the bitterness you sometimes get in olive oil," in addition to having "a haunting, nutty vanilla flavor" perfectly suited to curries, baked goods and sautés. Beyond its culinary appeal, coconut oil is becoming an increasingly popular ingredient in the kitchens of the health-conscious thanks to a few more reasons.

Because of its high lauric acid content, coconut oil is a quite popular replacement for other more dangerous alternatives such as trans fats. Whereas these worse options tend to raise LDL counts, coconut oil does the exact opposite. It doesn't just stop at lowering LDL either; some researchers believe that coconut oil also contributes to an increase in HDL throughout the system.

Lauric acid is also thought to assist in combating harmful viruses and bacteria. Research confirms the bevy of benefits offered to users of coconut oil. A study from Tehran asserted its beneficial impact on cardiovascular health, and another out of India concluded that coconut oil improved one's cholesterol balance as well as their antioxidant levels.

As if that were not enough, coconut oil is also marketed as a product for skin and hair care, and is thought to be effective in assisting with weight loss and digestion.

Chapter Seventeen:

Unlike the unfortunate stigma carried by fats, proteins have long been heralded for their association with all things masculine – not to mention that protein is the second of the two major building blocks of the human diet. After all, who among us can forget the famous scene of Rocky chugging raw eggs while training for the big fight? Fortunately protein is also available in slightly more palatable forms, such as a thick juicy steak and delicious natural protein shakes – some of which are even vegan friendly!

Apart from making you look manly while ingesting it, protein serves a number of purposes. It is found in every different kind of cell, and is the most plentiful molecule within the human body besides water. Our bodies need protein to build bone, skin, hair, nails and cell membranes, and to manufacture blood, hormones, neurochemicals, immune cells and enzymes. That's because proteins contain amino acids, nutrients that provide our bodies with a constant supply of nitrogen and sulphur. Nitrogen and sulfur are also essential to the ongoing growth, repair and detoxification of all our cells. In fact, nitrogen balance (the measure of how much nitrogen is retained as opposed to excreted) is the measurement researchers use to determine protein requirements.

Protein not only supports lean muscle mass, but without it, it would be impossible for tissues to regenerate after exercise, rendering all your efforts absolutely futile. Working out is tough enough as it is; to do so for naught will leave you singing a tune much sadder than the Beer Belly Blues.

How it Works

In order to function, protein is transported to the stomach, where the process of digestion breaks it down and makes its individual building blocks – amino acids – available to the body. The human body requires 22 amino acids in order to make more than 50,000 different proteins variations for optimal health. However, these are further classified into two separate categories: essential and non-essential. Essential amino acids, must be obtained through one's diet, as the body cannot manufacture them on its own, whereas non-essential amino acids can be synthesized naturally in the human body from available sources (i.e. essential amino acids or from other proteins).

Examples of non-essential amino acids include *glutamine*, which is marketed as a supplement for muscle growth (although under certain circumstances, such as a compromised immune system, glutamine can also be considered conditionally essential); *glycine*, which is sold as a sweetener and food additive; and *asparagine*, the first amino acid ever to be isolated in a laboratory setting (and also the reason that your pee smells funny after eating asparagus).

Some essential amino acids include *phenylalanine*, a main ingredient in aspartame (the artificial sweetener branded as NutraSweet and Equal); *tryptophan*, the chemical component frequently (and erroneously) blamed for causing drowsiness after eating turkey; and my personal favorite, *leucine*, which, along with *isoleucine* and *valine*, is classified as a *branched chain amino acid*.

The Real Deal with Essential and Nonessential

Even though researchers have discovered 22 standard amino acids, only 20 of these are directly encoded into our genes (DNA). As humans, we have the ability to manufacture 11 of the 20 amino acids – these are the non-essential ones – from each other or from other molecules and the other nine must be consumed in the diet – these are the essential ones.

Branched-Chain Amino Acids

Without making you feel like you are taking a biochemistry class, branched chain amino acids (or BCAAs) are amino acids featuring a chain with a branch. Okay, perhaps that is simplifying it a bit too much, as it just sounds like two-thirds of a recipe for a really tiny tire swing. Let's just skip to what they are all about.

BCAAS constitute over a third of the essential amino acids found in muscle proteins, and have been associated with a number of important phenomena. In August 2011, *Science Translational Medicine* published a study linking BCAAs to an improvement in the regulation of blood sugar levels, while another article printed in the January 2006 edition of *The*

Journal of Nutrition highlights the therapeutic values of BCAAs when used to treat patients with burns, trauma and sepsis.

Furthermore, as noted in an article published in a 2005 issue of the *Journal of Physiology*, leucine is the only amino acid shown to stimulate the body's production of muscle protein. This makes it particularly invaluable in counteracting the results of aging, as a leucine-rich diet can help to slow the natural decline in muscle tissue associated with the Beer Belly Blues. The success of such a plan was discussed by Brazilian researchers in the *Journal of the International Society of Sports Nutrition*, wherein they concluded that BCAA supplementation proved beneficial in dealing with exercise-based muscle damage, particularly in reducing muscle soreness. Theoretically this would allow for quicker recovery times between workout sessions, allowing for a more intense exercise regimen in terms of both frequency and intensity and bolstering one's ability to combat the Beer Belly Blues via physical activity.

While BCAAs can be obtained through a number of dietary sources, certain foods carry higher levels of these specialized amino acids than others. For instance, valine is abundant in cottage cheese, whole grains, mushrooms and peanuts. Isoleucine can be found in many meats, fish and cheeses. Beans, brewer's yeast, brown rice, caseinate and corn all contain comparably high levels of leucine. In addition, high levels of all three are present in both egg and whey protein.

BCAA's and the Beer Belly

The amount of muscle we carry dictates how many calories we are able to burn each day (referred to as our resting metabolic rate). The problem is, when people go on the majority of unbalanced diets – especially without incorporating weight-bearing exercise – they often lose muscle mass. This is also one of the primary reasons so many dieters hit a weight-loss plateau where fat loss comes to a sudden halt.

In order to maintain an efficient metabolism, especially while dieting, it is imperative to ensure adequate protein intake with special emphasis on the branched-chain amino acids. Research presented in the *Journal of Nutrition* showed that by adding proteins (approximately 125 grams/day) known for their high amounts of branched-chain amino acids, people were able to maintain muscle mass while reducing body fat during weight loss. The study looked at protein foods (125 grams each day for 10 weeks consisting of

10 ounces of meat – including one beef serving – as well as three servings of low-fat milk or cheese) that provided optimal levels of the branched-chain amino acid, leucine. Dr. Donald Layman, professor of nutrition at the University of Illinois where the study was conducted, said, "Traditionally, people have built a diet around low-fat foods, instead of high-quality protein foods. Study participants following the moderately high protein plan were twice as effective in maintaining lean muscle mass."

A Better *Whey* to Beat the Beer Belly Blues

If you've ever been into any sort of health-food or nutritional store, chances are you are familiar with whey protein. Those big plastic tubs are more or less visually synonymous with working out, as it seems everyone from the moderately health-conscious to the most hardcore of bodybuilders swear by their powdery contents. Certainly that many sweaty exercise enthusiasts couldn't be wrong, so what's the deal?

Formed from the byproducts of the cheese manufacturing process, whey contains all the soluble items left behind once milk coagulates. Its proteins are then isolated, thus leaving behind the powdery diet supplement so many have come to know and love. There are two primary varieties, known as concentrate and isolate, which cater to the different expectations of the user. The concentrate form offers comparably lower levels of fat and cholesterol but higher levels of bioactive compounds and carbohydrates (including the primary milk sugar, lactose); the isolate form is lower in bioactive compounds but also has been removed of its fat and lactose content and is thereby easier to metabolize (i.e. it works quicker and better) but tends to be more expensive.

Apart from the heightened capacity to build muscle, the use of whey protein is thought to help reduce the risk of heart disease and cancer. Additionally, an article published in the *Journal of Nutritional Biochemistry* asserts that the especially high leucine content of whey protein makes it an excellent stimulant of muscle repair and recovery.

Don't forget, a general loss of muscle mass, tone and strength are also symptoms of both the Beer Belly Blues and simply getting old. While lower testosterone levels will make it harder for the body to build lean muscle mass and maintain strength, the loss of protein will produce similar results, which is also where whey protein can help.

With advanced age (I'm talking over 40 here), it becomes more difficult for the body to absorb protein, which can lead to a number of issues including lowered immunity, slower healing times, and the loss of muscle mass. Some proteins are absorbed slowly by the body while others, like whey, are absorbed rapidly. In one study conducted by researchers in Europe on elderly men comparing the absorption of slowly digested proteins versus rapidly absorbed ones, participants absorbed whey compared to other proteins such as casein (the primary protein found in milk). The whey protein was very effective at preventing muscle loss and strength in the elderly subjects even though their protein absorption was somewhat hindered by age. There is no reason not to think that high-quality whey protein supplements couldn't help reduce the loss of muscle mass due to lower testosterone levels.

The research is clear: properly processed whey protein formulas are able to help combat symptoms of the Beer Belly Blues, such as maintaining prostate health, reducing cancer risk, and reversing muscle loss and reduced bone strength. But on top of helping combat the common and sometimes deadly symptoms of the Beer Belly Blues, whey protein also appears to dramatically improve overall longevity, at least if animal studies are any indication. In a six-month study conducted on rats who (in human terms) were aged from 55 to 80, an all-whey protein diet significantly enhanced survival rates while improving the overall health of heart and liver tissue.

While it seems that more health benefits of whey protein are being discovered every day, one thing is abundantly clear: For men looking to combat the Beer Belly Blues and improve overall health, including whey protein in their daily diet is a win-win situation.

The Alpha Male

Let's face it: trying to find a high-quality whey protein formula these days can be daunting. First off, there are too many formulas to count, and all of them claim to have the best protein around! So what should you really look for when it comes to whey protein? Look for high levels of something called *alphalactalbumin* or alpha, for short. The "alpha" portion of whey happens to contain the exact amino acids that are found in the most important protein regarding human growth and repair – mother's breast milk. In fact, approximately 33 percent of breast milk consists of this imperative protein structure.

High-alpha whey isolates have been shown in numerous human studies to be highly effective in improving the efficiency of exercise and decreasing excess body fat. Aside from this, these high alpha whey isolates help to improve brain performance in people who are easily affected by stress by increasing the amount of brain tryptophan and serotonin (the feel-good neurochemical). If that wasn't enough, a study appearing in the *American Journal of Clinical Nutrition* showed that these proteins were also able to improve sleep patterns and increase morning alertness in participants with mild sleep problems.

Testosterone and Protein

Aside from its role in helping to regenerate the body's ability to build vital muscle tissue – which in its own right is a testosterone-supporting act – protein also indirectly helps to elevate testosterone levels by lowering the testosterone-binding protein SHBG. In the January 2000 issue of the *Journal of Clinical Endocrinology & Metabolism*, researchers from the University of Massachusetts Medical School published their findings from an investigation into the link between diet and SHBG levels: "The lower the protein intake, the higher the concentration of SHBG. This … indicates that protein intake can be an important control of SHBG level." Thinking back a few chapters, you might remember that lower SHBG levels mean higher levels of free testosterone, something we here at the Beer Belly Blues Headquarters officially classify as a "good thing."

Prehistoric Protein

Almost everyone has heard the saying, "You are what you eat." This statement is only partly true. We are not only what we eat, but more importantly, we are also what our ancestors ate. And guess what? According to archaeological, anthropological, physiological and fossil evidence, our ancestors ate protein, and lots of it. We have evolved to run best on the same foods as our prehistoric ancestors – and their diet consisted of at least 30 percent protein.

Of course, the protein our ancestors ate was a little different from much of the protein we consume today. Early man consumed protein from lean game meats, which also contained the essential fatty acids I spoke about in the last chapter, not to mention many other nutrients we are lacking in our contemporary diets. Other research indicates that we were predominantly hunters and then gatherers. It is interesting that the research also indicates that our early ancestors were much healthier than the people of the agricultural revolution, who consumed a diet high in carbohydrates.

Chapter Eighteen:
////////////////// **Ultimate Male Supplements**

We all know how the old saying goes: "An apple a day keeps the doctor away." Having grown up with phrases like this, we likely just take them for granted rather than giving them any sort of critical thought. Some of these phrases, upon further scrutiny, prove to be false – nothing more than old wives' tales that serve no purpose other than to perpetuate themselves: a watched pot will, in fact, boil, and neither your luck nor your stomach will suffer for seven years after breaking a mirror or swallowing chewing gum. The ones that do ring true, like the example above, are worth keeping in mind. After all, maintaining one's health through naturally obtained nutrients (such as organic apples) is not only an effective way to cut down on the need for doctor's visits, but also a much preferable course of action to taking the prescription medications you would receive otherwise. As they say, the answer isn't always at the bottom of a bottle (of pills, in this instance). In fact, the answer is much closer than you might think.

Thanks to a combination of new advances into natural remedies and a veritable treasure trove of time-tested information, it is more possible than ever to preserve and improve your health through holistic means. The growing popularity of such products can be witnessed both in the proliferation of the specialty stores that carry them, and their emergence on the shelves of more traditional retailers. More importantly, this isn't due to any hidden financial agenda, as these products lack the backing of the big pharmaceutical corporations that have made household names of so many pills and powders. Instead, many of the natural remedies are gaining steam for one simple reason: they work. When taken properly, natural supplements offer all the benefits of their synthetic counterparts without the considerable drawbacks of side effects, making them an essential part of one's day-to-day wellness regimen.

While there are all-natural supplements and nutrients suggested for the treatment of every ailment from the flu to foot fungus, here are a few that are particularly relevant to those going through the Beer Belly Blues, and of especial interest to anyone happening to be bothered by our less-than-ideal pal ED.

Testosterone-Supporting Nutrients

To recap what we have learned so far: testosterone is good – very good in fact. It helps regulate a number of our vital functions and its natural tendency to diminish along with aging is what ushers in the Beer Belly Blues. Therefore, maintenance of testosterone levels is absolutely a priority, especially when it can be done through healthy, natural and research-proven means, as are the following items.

Peruvian Maca – Found high in the Andes mountain range in Peru, *Lepidium meyenii* is a perennial root vegetable with a number of medicinal properties (some of which we will be revisiting later). Similar to a radish or turnip, maca has seen more than 2,000 years of use dating back to the indigenous people of the area who employed it as a foodstuff, a form of currency and an aphrodisiac. While still used for the first purpose (much less so for the second), maca remains even more relevant to the third, especially in terms of this text. While maca has yet to be tied directly to the increased production of testosterone, its unique combination of nutrients is thought to have an overall salutary effect on the endocrine system, thus allowing for the optimization of its functions, including the manufacture and binding of hormones.

Chrysin (with Bioperine) – If you can think back a few chapters, you might recall the problems posed by aromatase, the enzyme used in synthesizing estrogen from testosterone. If you are having trouble with the memory, just think back to "man boobs." Yes, I thought you might remember aromatase as being a very, very bad thing (at least when left unchecked). Fortunately, chrysin is around to help prevent a future in which we need to choose a T-shirt based on how well it accentuates our cleavage. It is a naturally occurring flavoring agent found in both blue passion flower and honeycomb, and is popular with those undergoing rigorous strength training (such as athletes or bodybuilders) for its renowned ability to keep aromatase levels (as well as our cup sizes) in check.

While research has found that there may be difficulty in absorbing chrysin into the bloodstream, it has also found a natural way to improve results. Bioperine, a component of black pepper and long pepper, is thought to help the body in deriving the maximum benefit possible from chrysin when the two are taken together. It does so by slowing down the process of metabolism, thereby enhancing the bioavailability of certain substances, including the active agents in chrysin.

Stinging Nettle Root – The medicinal use of stinging nettle root can be traced all the way back to the 10th century, when it was included in a pagan manual called the *Nine Herbs Charm*. Since then, stinging nettle root has been used as a folk remedy for a maladies such as rheumatism, arthritis and dandruff. It has also been researched as a potential tool in the treatment of benign prostatic hyperplasia (BPH), which we touched on briefly in a previous chapter (hint: It was the one about the prostate).

It is also popular in soups and in a couple of forms of beverage, including a sweetened tea-like version and a type of beer.

Those also wishing to increase their levels of free testosterone take stinging nettle root. It works by preemptively occupying the binding sites of SHBG, which has a tendency to bind with free testosterone if not otherwise engaged.

See, I told you this was all important information that would pay off as we went!

Indole 3 Carbinol (I3C) – I3C is the byproduct of the breakdown of *glucosinolate glucobrassicin*, a nutrient found in high concentrations in the leafy green cruciferous plants such as cabbage, bok choy and broccoli. It has been noted for its ability to convert estrogens from a form particularly deleterious to those in the midst of the Beer Belly Blues (*16-alpha hydroxyestrone*) into other harmless ones. In addition to this application in the pursuit of higher testosterone levels, it has also been used in the treatment of lupus and human *papillomavirus*.

Prostate-Protecting Nutrients

If you consider your "unit" the quarterback of Team Down There, then the prostate would certainly qualify as the offensive line: less glamorous, for sure, but absolutely integral to the function of the entire squad. In order to keep up its good work, your prostate needs just as much attention as your MVP, as without it he'd be nowhere.

Beta-Sitosterol – Operating in a function we are by now quite familiar with, beta-Sitosterol lowers cholesterol levels in order to improve one's overall well-being. Found in pecans, pumpkin seeds and standardized extracts of saw palmetto, it primarily does so by impairing the intestine's ability to absorb cholesterol. It has been investigated in conjunction with prostatic cancer treatments, and has also been identified as a useful aid in cases of BPH.

Flower Pollen – Probably the most familiar item on the list, flower pollen nevertheless offers some surprising health benefits for the prostate. First off, it interacts with hormones known to cause BPH (again!) when found in excessive levels, preventing them from reproducing or binding properly. Flower pollen is also thought to reduce inflammation, a main source of the discomfort stemming from prostate-related disorders. Finally, it is known to relax smooth muscles such as those found in the prostate. Undue tension can result in contraction near the neck of the bladder, which in turn makes urinating problematic. By relaxing them, flower pollen eases the process.

Selenium (selenomethionine) – With an atomic number (34) and a chemical symbol (Se) all to itself, selenium might seem less like a health supplement than an origin of some comic hero's superpowers. While comparably rare in nature, selenium is in fact an essential trace nutrient derived from such sources as Brazil nuts, tuna and crab. In a study designed to investigate the effects of selenium supplementation on the development of various forms of cancer, it was found that patients with higher levels of selenium developed fewer cases of prostate cancer.

Bioavailable Zinc – According to the *Journal of Nutrition*, zinc is considered a nutrient of "exceptional biologic and public health importance." An essential mineral, zinc deficiency affects an estimated two billion people worldwide, especially those in developing nations, and can result in stunted growth and fertility problems. While it can also be fatally poisonous in excess, zinc taken in the proper amount can prove vital in ensuring prostate health. Studies show that zinc is essential for the maintenance of healthy testosterone levels and men who have low levels of this master mineral usually find their testosterone lowering along with it. Aside from this, it is currently being researched for its astounding ability to target and kill prostate cancer cells.

Libido-Enhancing Nutrients

While the previous few supplements will aid you in your ability to walk the walk, these next few will make sure you are equally willing to talk the talk. After all, owning the equipment only adds up to so much when you lack the desire to use it. Even a Rolls-Royce is just an expensive lawn ornament when you've got no one interesting in driving it. These next few natural remedies can help get you itching to be behind the wheel again, so to speak.

Peruvian Maca – Even though I mentioned this one in the Testosterone-Supporting Nutrients section above, it is definitely worth mentioning again, as libido enhancement is one of maca's most spoken-about qualities. Studies published in *Forsch Komplementmed, Andrologia* (don't even try pronouncing it), and the *Asian Journal of Andrology* confirm that maca offers a number of benefits to the reproductive system, including improving both libido and semen quality in terms of volume and sperm motility and function. All around, maca is a superstar when it comes to putting the schwing back in your thing!

Tongkat Ali – Native to the area encompassing Malaysia and Thailand, tongkat ali is a flowering plant known for its medicinal qualities, as well as its bitter flavor. While known to scientists as *Eurycoma longifolia*, according to the journal *Nature*, it is better-known for being a natural alternative to Viagra. In addition to increasing sexual desire, researchers have found it to be effective in raising testosterone levels and reversing the effects of estrogen on testosterone production.

Epimedium – Horny Goat Weed: this nickname should say it all. Horny goat weed originated as an ancient Chinese cure allegedly discovered by a goat farmer whose flock got into a patch. *Icariin*, the active ingredient in horny goat weed, not only relaxes smooth muscle tissue in a way similar to flower pollen, but also acts as a PDE5 inhibitor. As you might recall from the last chapter, that is the exact same chemical function that is the basis for the three major ED drugs. Simply put, it is as close to a natural prescription as you will get.

Conclusion

Although the nutrients listed above have been validated both through studies and anecdotal reports, it is important to understand that not all products on the market contain the right extracts or dosages of each one. Aside from this, dosages may vary depending on each individual case, so speaking to a naturally trained health professional can help determine which ones and what dosages are best for you (and your unit). Having said this, there also are products available that contain synergistic blends of these nutrients, which could end up saving you big money in the long run. Finally, properly designed libido-enhancing supplements take time to work – sometimes up to a month – so be patient and enjoy the results!

Chapter Nineteen:
Don't Exercise – Biocize

Whether you want to believe it or not, we were all given a miraculous machine capable of moving us around at peak proficiency. In youth, the human body is amazing indeed. Given the proper training and fuel, it can be programmed to achieve remarkable feats of speed, agility, flexibility and strength. If you don't believe me, all you have to do is eavesdrop on a couple of over-the-hill weight lifters boasting about how much weight they could lift, how much mobility they had and how little pain they felt in their younger years.

Unfortunately too many of us never give a second thought to the downward inevitability that a sedentary lifestyle eventually brings. We ignore the fact that by retirement age nearly two-thirds of the population will have lost at least one-third of their lean body mass (muscle, bone and organs) and gained the rest in – you guessed it – lard. Who cares how much lean body mass you lose? No one really wants to look like Arnold what's-his-name anyway. The fact is lean body mass also brings with it confidence, health and vitality (all of which are fundamental to healthy testosterone levels). Muscle strength and your cardio-respiratory rate become limiting factors as you age so that simple things you take for granted when you're young, such as getting out of a chair or walking to the store and carrying a few groceries, can now become a chore.

Almost everything we do on a daily basis requires muscle strength and our vital capacity – the ability to take in and utilize oxygen from the air we breathe. Lung performance usually reaches its maximum around 16 years of age and then declines by about 1 percent a year thereafter, so that by the time we are around 60 years of age, we may only have two-thirds to one-half of the capacity we once had. Losing our vital capacity can result in much more than needing to take a few extra breaths. It can lead to serious heart conditions and a greater susceptibility to pneumonia and other kinds of infections. If you've been ignoring the facts until this point, by now you must realize the vast importance in both retaining lean body mass (muscle tissue and strength) as well as holding on to your vital capacity as you get older.

While other lifestyle-management techniques such as diet and stress management are important, nothing comes close to physical activity in terms of having an impact on overall health, and on testosterone levels as well. Noting its importance, a *Journal of American Medical Association* article suggested that "Every US adult should accumulate 30 minutes or more of moderate-intensity physical activity on most, preferably all, days of the week." Apart from improving the health of the body as a whole, which allows for the increased functionality of all systems (which happen to include those responsible for testosterone production), the right exercise has been shown to have a more direct link to testosterone health. A 1996 study examined the effect of exercise on the sex hormone levels of otherwise sedentary men ranging in age from 66 to 76. While in good health apart from their inactivity, periods of exercise were shown to raise serum testosterone levels by 39 percent, and boosted their all-important free testosterone counts by 23 percent.

It's All In Your Mind

A study published in the journal *Health Psychology* showed that the myriad benefits of exercise could be attributed in part to a person's self-confidence. The emotional high that people experience from physical activity depends in part on what they believe they are capable of, or what researchers call the exercise "self-efficacy." The study showed that the higher a person's self-belief, the more likely he or she is to feel emotional benefits from regular exercise. Dr. McAuley, lead researcher in the study, suggests that enhancing self-belief can improve any exercise experience, at least emotionally. People who believe they are incapable of exercising might feel themselves getting tired, reach their limit earlier or drop out of an exercise program, while those with a higher belief system would actually feel great about the experience. It all starts in your head – if you think you can, you most likely will!

I am sure you haven't forgotten how low testosterone can negatively affect mood and lead to major bouts of depression, and in turn how depression (and low testosterone) can lead to ED. Well it turns out that proper exercise can elicit powerful mood-lifting changes. In fact, a major study performed at Duke University Medical Center in England showed that certain exercises can be just as effective as some of the most prescribed medications when it comes to alleviating major depression. The study looked at 156 elderly patients diagnosed with major depressive disorder over a 16-week period. The participants were assigned to three separate groups: Group 1 exercised but had no antidepressants; group 2 took anti-depressant medication with no exercise; and group 3 took antidepressant medication combined with exercise. To the amazement of the researchers, all three groups showed remarkably similar improvements in their depressive states following the 16-week trial. This study, as well as numerous others, proves that exercise should be considered a viable alternative to medication when it comes to one of our most treated disorders of aging.

Introducing Biocize

Biocize exercise is a training concept born of the realization that many of the changes in health status that have been deemed the normal result of aging (i.e. the Beer Belly Blues) are actually the result of a long-standing sedentary lifestyle coupled with poor diet, excess stress and lack of deep sleep.

Research indicates that activity in the later years of life (middle age) is strongly correlated with the level of a senior citizen's independence. So if you are one of those independent types, this is one more incentive to get moving. In essence, movement, strength and flexibility are among the most powerful tools for a liberated, independent, Beer-Belly-Blues-FREE life.

How was Biocize Developed?

Biocize exercise was developed after researching the most effective exercise strategies (including timing, duration, hormonal elevations and nutrient partitioning) for their positive affects on one's biological age from a hormonal perspective. After all, hormones are the key cellular messengers, and losing key messages (through the decline of certain fundamental hormones such as testosterone) as we age is one of the biological markers of aging itself.

How does Biocize Work?

Biocize is all about short duration and high impact. In other words, life is about living, as opposed to spending hours in a gym. Get in – get out – get on with your life.

By understanding a few key principles about exercise, it is possible to begin reaping the benefits of this revolutionary workout regimen today. There are, however, a few things you need to familiarize yourself with first.

Aerobic exercise is a form of exercise that tends to be of the low-impact, long-duration variety, such as walking or jogging. It is intended to stimulate the process of energy generation via the process of oxygen consumption, which is fairly easy to remember considering that "aerobic" translates to "living with air." It improves the respiratory function, strengthens the heart, burns fat (although it takes a long, long time to notice any of the effects of this type of training), and builds lean muscle.

Anaerobic exercise, on the other hand, consists of short-burst exercises designed to build speed and power, such as lifting weights or sprinting. Whereas aerobic exercise relies on oxygen for energy, anaerobic exercise relies on the development of the fast-twitch muscle fibers in order to deliver these quickly needed energy resources.

Prolonged periods of both sorts of exercise can lead to the build-up of **lactic acid**, a chemical most often confused with the muscle soreness felt after strenuous activity (actually, lactic acid is a very beneficial chemical when it comes to stimulating the right hormones through exercise). The intensity of anaerobic exercise can be quantified in terms of its lactic threshold (LT), or the point at which the body starts producing lactic acid faster than it can absorb it, allowing it to accumulate in the blood stream.

Gaining Muscle and Losing Fat with Biocize

Most people think that aerobic types of exercise are the best for long-term fat loss. Unfortunately, they're wrong in this approach. Unless you're planning on getting a flat, your main objective is to get rid of the spare tire. If you commit yourself solely to aerobic training, then you will be carrying around the spare for a lot longer than you'd like. Studies show that too much cardio performed in the absence of resistance training can be detrimental to long-term fat loss. Cardio itself is not the enemy. The problem lies in the amount and intensity of the cardio activity. The truth is, too much cardio exercise is detrimental to your metabolic engine, muscle. Research has confirmed that cardio activity cannot maintain muscle mass on its own.

In a landmark study published in the *American Journal of Cardiology*, aerobic training was compared to aerobic with resistance (weight) training. Two groups had to complete a 10-week exercise program of 75 minutes. One group completed 75 minutes of aerobic exercise twice a week, while the other completed 40 minutes of aerobics plus 35 minutes of weight training. The time spent training was identical. At the end of the study, the aerobics group showed an 11 percent increase in endurance, but no increase in their strength. The group that completed the combination of aerobics plus weight training showed a massive 109 percent increase in their endurance, and a 21-43 percent increase in their overall strength. There are many other studies that further prove the theory that resistance training combined with low-impact cardio is superior to either one alone.

Join the Resistance

Exercises such as walking at a fast pace will do wonders for your vital capacity, but unfortunately it won't reverse the two top biomarkers of the Beer Belly Blues – loss of lean body mass and body-fat accumulation. In order to rebuild the old muscle tissue with new stronger fibers and incinerate the fat, you must work out in an anaerobic fashion. Anaerobic exercise creates intensity sufficient enough to ensure that the muscles cannot receive enough oxygen transfer. As the muscles strain to work in this environment, extra lactic acid is released – in other words, the more vigorous the exercise, the higher the lactic-acid production. Newer research confirms that lactic acid benefits the heart and also helps to cleanse our systems by binding to and removing toxic metals that accumulate over time. The more intense the activity, the higher your lactate threshold becomes, allowing you to exercise with a great deal more intensity than you previously could.

This anaerobic environment and the lactate threshold help to stimulate growth hormone and testosterone, which, as you are now well aware, are needed for building new muscle mass. Growth hormone and testosterone are responsible for the hypertrophy (increased size and density) of muscle cells, as well as the repair of micro-tears in the muscle tissue. Together they increase your anabolic metabolism (rebuild, repair and replace worn, damaged cells throughout the body). Nothing accomplishes this task better than a Biocize exercise program.

The Real Magic of Biocize Exercise

Another benefit of Biocize exercise lies in its ability to raise your metabolic rates (the rate at which you burn calories at rest) afterward. A great deal of this is due to the rise in anabolic (rebuild and repair) hormones testosterone and growth hormone, not only as you exercise, but approximately 15 minutes after the exercise is completed. As long as you don't blunt this metabolic increase by consuming high-carbohydrate energy drink (such as Gatorade®), in the absence of protein your body will have the ability to burn calories for many hours to come. As a matter of fact, one study showed that more than two-thirds of the fat-burning activity of high-intensity exercise takes place *after* the actual exercise sessions. This increase in fat-burning potential has been documented as lasting for more than 15 hours in highly trained athletes, and is believed to be due to the increased activity of a fat-releasing enzyme called *hormone-sensitive lipase* or HSL.

What's the Best Way to Biocize?

So which form of exercise is superior? This is something to ask yourself when trying to construct the ideal workout routine. If you've learned anything from the past few chapters, you will know that moderation in all things is key – meaning that a precise mixture of both seems to be the best in terms of maximum results for minimal efforts. *Let's face it, in today's hustle and bustle world, who has time to pursue two entirely different types of exercise?* In fact, most people barely feel as if they have enough time for any exercise at all. The beautiful part about Biocize is that you can combine your efforts and do both at once.

Over the last decade exercise physiologists have discovered that high-intensity interval training provides the best of both worlds, as it allows you to exercise both systems at once. This type of training – also referred to as Tabata Training, founded in Japan by Izumi Tabata – proves that super-high-intensity training over very short periods (as in 4-minute sets) elicits the greatest hormonal response (growth hormone and testosterone = results) in the least amount of time.

The basic outline of Biocize exercise via Tabata Training is as follows:

- **4 minutes** – each session (per exercise)
- **20 seconds** – duration of intense training
- **10 seconds** – rest period
- **8 sessions or sets** – in total

The beauty of 4-minute Biocize programs is that they can be applied to almost any exercise (as long as you adhere to proper form). If you use Biocize training techniques (short duration-high impact), you will be able to see better results in record time by improving both the aerobic and anaerobic system at the same time. As mentioned, newer research shows that a duration as short as 4 minutes can bring incredible results in record time. In a 1996 research study that tested the Tabata method as shown above (referred to as the IE1 protocol), against more traditional exercise methodologies, found that those using the IE1 protocol system gained not only more overall muscle mass, but also additional anaerobic benefits not seen in the traditional workout group. This is due in part to the cross-training's unique ability to allow the body to perform above its traditional lactate threshold for brief periods, which forces the body to regenerate in a more efficient manner.

The key to Biocize is to give your all during the all-out intense 20-second periods. In other words, you are only cheating yourself if you don't push it to the max each time. If you are performing the activity right, 4 minutes should feel like an eternity, but trust me when I say that once you are done, you will feel like a million bucks, and as soon as you see how quick the results will come, you'll only want to push it harder the next time around.

Another Biocize Option When It Comes to Cardio

When it comes to cardio-type exercising alone using the Biocize principles, there is another option to consider (also referred to as Peak 8 by Dr. Joseph Mercola) – especially if you enjoy working out a little longer. This option only applies to cardio training as it is very difficult and potentially problematic to incorporate it into resistance exercise (i.e. weight training). The total duration of this other option is 20 minutes broken up into 8 sessions of 30-second all-out effort followed by minute and a half rest periods. This works quite well when performing exercises such as walking at a fast pace, being on an elliptical machine or a recumbent bike, etc.

The equation is as follows:

- **3 minute warm-up** – i.e. walking at a fast pace

- **30 seconds** of all out effort (as in sprinting or peddling as fast as possible)

- **1 minute, 30-second** rest period (as in moving at a pace that is slow enough to bring your heart rate to normal and allow you to breath normally again)

- **3 minute** cool-down
- **8 sessions** or sets – in total

Core Biocize Resistance Training

Normally there is no set repetition range when it comes to effective weight training. Some experts believe 4-6 reps per exercise builds the most muscle, others believe that 8-10 reps is the best way to go, and still others believe you should strive for 15 and up. When it comes to Biocize exercise, we aren't interested in what is normally carried out during a well-designed exercise program. Instead we are interested only in getting the best hormonal bang for your buck.

It turns out that higher-intensity weight training affects growth hormone and testosterone response much better than low-intensity weight training. What does high intensity equate to? According to exercise physiologists, approximately 70 percent of your maximal lifting capacity will induce a threefold increase in growth hormone levels, while lifting at 85 percent of your max will quadruple it. In a 1991 Pennsylvania State University study performed by Dr. William Kraemer and associates, the best rep sequence for maximum growth hormone output for both men and women was 8-10 reps with a 1-minute rest in between.

If you are not interested in performing the all out 4-minute Biocize training methodologies and are looking for something a little more routine but with greater results, then try the above method of lifting weights or using resistance bands for 8-10 reps followed by 1-minute rest intervals for 3-4 sets in total. If you follow this type of a strategy when performing resistance exercises, you will be adhering – at least in part – to the Biocize philosophy. For maximum hormonal effect, try performing multi-joint or compound exercises to facilitate the greatest number of muscle fibers. Compound exercises include those that target more than one muscle group, such as a bench press (upper body) or squats (lower body). I'll present more information related to Biocize exercises in Part III.

So, now that you are aware of the optimum sequence of resistance training needed to elicit beneficial results while following Biocize exercise, exactly how much weight training is enough? In order to answer this question you first have to understand that resistance exercise is somewhat stressful to the body (which is why taking regular breaks from this form of exercising is wise). The good news is that a little stress helps make the body stronger (not to mention more effective at letting go of stubborn fat), but too much can cause a drastic increase in the muscle-wasting hormone cortisol. Depending on your activity level, soon after 45 minutes the levels of cortisol and free radicals rise to the point where recovery from the exercise can become blunted. Cortisol is responsible for stealing valuable nitrogen from muscle tissue, and then converting that muscle into extra energy. The more cortisol produced, the harder it is to get rid of and the worse off you are. Talk about a waste of valuable time spent exercising! So the rule of thumb is no more than 45 minutes of the weight-training portion of your Biocize workout.

So there you have it. Who says you have to spend hours in a gym to get into the best shape of your life? In addition to being a more effective training system, Biocize is also more time efficient. Biocizing means less time spent sweating in the gym and more time outside enjoying the better things life has to offer. So don't just exercise, Biocize!

Chapter Twenty:
////////////////////// **Booze, Babies and Testosterone**

Much like the Apocalypse relies on the Four Horseman as harbingers of doom, the Beer Belly Blues has a pair of Killer B's that can spell trouble for your testosterone. Though both occupy prominent roles in the day-to-day lives of many, if not most, members of society, both booze and babies complicate matters by contributing whole new sets of risk factors to your already hectic life. Without knowing how to properly manage these new distractions, it is entirely possible to lose track of yourself as well as any progress you have made, or would otherwise be capable of making, toward finding the ideal you. However, by becoming aware of the dangers posed by the Killer B's, it entirely possible to make the appropriate accommodations necessary to incorporate them within your plan for total wellness.

Booze

Let's face it – sometimes nothing in life beats a good, strong drink. Whether it's a cold beer after a long day's work, a glass of fine scotch to celebrate a recent promotion, or a frozen fruity beverage enjoyed in the shade of a sandy beach, the right beverage can help to make a bad day good and a good day great. Unfortunately, alcohol is not without its drawbacks. I suppose calling this period the "Beer Belly Blues" was somewhat of a giveaway regarding some of our priorities during this trying stage of life, as many of us find our T-shirt inexplicably shrinking in direct proportion to how many of these liquid cure-alls we have imbibed. However, the role alcohol plays in our diet and lifestyle may be more complicated than you think.

Booze and Body Fat

Contrary to what you might think, the predominant cause of the dietary problems attributed to alcohol consumption is not a simple matter of calories. While it is true that adult beverages contain a high level of what are considered to be empty calories – that is, calories without the redeeming nutritional value of fats and proteins – it is not so much their quantity as their quality that proves troublesome. These empty calories are exceedingly easy for the body to break down and use for energy, making them the no-brainer solution for a machine that maximizes its efficiency by following the path of least-possible resistance. Rather than toil away at metabolizing the more complex, nutrient-laden calorie sources, the body stores these away for later use.

Much in the same way those boxes you're planning on sorting through when you have a free minute tend to pile up in the attic and garage, these excess calories hang around in the form of unattractive body fat – primarily in the belly area. This process was tested by researchers from the University of California, who studied the metabolism of men within half an hour of consuming two alcoholic drinks. While the beverages themselves only contained approximately 90 calories apiece, their effects were considerably much larger – the men's ability to convert body fat into energy declined by an astounding 73 percent for a several-hour period.

Booze and the Bummers

In you have ever had a truly awful hangover – the pounding head, the twisted stomach, inability to process even the slightest amount of light or sound than anything short of nuclear war – then you know what a deterrent alcohol can be to any sort of activity, productive or otherwise. As a depressant, alcohol naturally suppresses motivation, reducing the urge to stay on target with such tasks as exercising and adhering to a strict diet. About the only thing drinking does encourage outside of making silly late-night phone calls or drunk-texting, is the tendency to snack, wreaking further havoc on your total wellness plan. Even if you manage to retain the dedication necessary to work out, too much alcohol may render the efforts useless, as excess drinking increases production of cortisol, a stress hormone capable of breaking down muscle tissue and thus diminishing the body's ability to burn calories.

Booze and Testosterone

Thinking back to the chapter regarding cholesterol, you might recall that cholesterol is not only necessary for the production of testosterone, but also that it is produced predominately in the liver (if not, feel free to go back and check. I won't tell anyone). As this is also the location where alcohol is metabolized –being turned first into a highly reactive substance called *acetaldehyde*, then into a compound called *acetic acid* (more commonly known as vinegar) – it shouldn't come as much of a surprise that one might have an effect on the other. A large number of the health problems associated with drinking target the liver, including cancer and cirrhosis. By impeding the liver's function, drinking has a direct negative impact on the body's ability to produce testosterone.

The journal *Alcohol* suggested that just one night of drinking could lead to an entire day's worth of generally lowered testosterone levels. Furthermore, acetaldehyde, in addition to being responsible free-radical damage and those miserable hangovers, is known to be a very effective testosterone inhibitor.

Babies

If for no other reason, babies would appear on this list for their amazing ability to make you want to drink. They're up till all hours, constantly making a racket, screaming incoherently for something you can't understand. Basically it's like living with your college roommate all over again, except this one has an excuse for when he can't make it to the bathroom in time. Sleepless nights can take a toll on anyone, and no matter how precious your overnight companion might be, this will eventually wear on you. A body cannot function optimally unless it is well rested, and it is tough to rest with a two-foot-high teakettle in the room beside you, constantly threatening to boil over. However, it's more than just being overtired that is threatening your testosterone levels.

In a study published in the 2011 edition of *Hormones and Behavior*, researchers evaluated the link between the noises created by babies (both sounds of distress, such as crying, and neutral/positive ones such as cooing, feeding, etc.) and the testosterone levels of the men who hear them. Even though the noises were played from a recording, scientists found they were still just as effective as the real thing. They theorized it was possible that the decrease in testosterone was a natural effort to bolster the brain and body's nurturing functions.

Researchers have found other links between testosterone loss and the mere presence of babies, howling or otherwise. A study of 624 young men in the Philippines found that men's testosterone levels tended to peak while searching for a female partner, but dropped between 26 and 34 percent upon becoming fathers. Scientists have theorized this is a response to changes in psychology regarding new social priorities, triggered by the release of bonding hormones such as *oxytocin* – the same hormone a woman pumps out that makes her want to cuddle after making love. The effect is not limited to babies, however, as it is fairly well-documented that unmarried men average higher levels of free testosterone than do their married counterparts.

Dealing With the Killer B's

Though there are some differences and some similarities between the two situations listed above, their main connection between the two is stress. While yes, it is possible to drink for other reasons – celebrations, for instance – stress can specifically lead to problematic drinking. Having one "just to calm the nerves" can easily turn into one "just for a pick me up" and then another one "just to face the day." Bars are also a favorite location for escapism, as they seem to be one of the last sanctuaries in which you can hide from the turmoil of everyday life – not to mention bond with a few buddies over a pint or two.

Babies also elevate stress levels because caring for an entirely new person is quite a step up from the customary workload of trying to take care of yourself. From remembering to bring the diaper bag to having to find not one but two matching pairs of socks before leaving the house, babies add an unexpected amount of hassle to your already hectic days. But rather than handling this by turning to the bottle (in more ways than one!), there are some very effective and simple ways to manage your own stress. Here are a few.

Avoid unnecessary stress – This can include stressful people, situations and issues. Sure, it might not be possible to totally avoid your newborn or your spouse, but dealing with them is certainly easier when you don't exhaust yourself yelling at the person at the grocery store trying to slip through the Ten-Items-or-Less lane with eleven tins of cat food.

Alter the situation – If you cannot avoid the situation entirely, learn to address it productively. Communicate your feelings in an assertive manner, but be willing to compromise. If it seems hopeless, reevaluate whether or not this situation is vital to your life and how it could otherwise be avoided.

Accept what you can't change – No matter how proactive you are, sometimes things are just unwinnable. Keep your chin up, remember it's not the end of the world, and look for the silver lining.

Value R & R – Even the most well-oiled machines need their downtime. In the grueling world of 24/7 business, it may seem tough to find downtime, but make it a priority. Apart from the obvious joy of leisure time, it will give your mind the opportunity to pull back and assess things from a different point of view, perhaps giving you the fresh perspective you need.

Stay healthy – It may seem obvious, but maintaining a healthy body is the best way to maintain a healthy body. The schedule and discipline it takes to stay in shape through exercise and dieting carries over into other aspects of life. Time spent focusing on how to better yourself is time that can't be wasted worrying yourself silly or worsening your well-being.

BONUS CHAPTER:

////////////// **The Unsung Hero - Appreciating Your Better Half**

So far we have spent a lot of time exploring the ways in which we can better ourselves, making sure we are absolutely the best we can be – becoming the Ultimate Male. Assuming, at least for the moment, that we have all this information well in hand and are on the way to achieving our ideal status, it would seem reasonable to take a moment to give back to those around us. After all, no man is an island. We receive a great amount of support from those around us, especially during the most trying moments of the Beer Belly Blues, and in doing so we put our loved ones through plenty.

While yes, the quest to make ourselves the best we can be is at least partially for their benefit, that's like buying your wife a bowling ball in your size with your own name engraved on it – no matter how well you gift-wrap it, it still doesn't count as a present for her. Our better halves deserve something more, which is why we are going to take this opportunity to add a few tips for better pleasing them, ensuring you will come out as a better whole.

Honor Her

Simply put, remember to show some R-E-S-P-E-C-T. Your wife or girlfriend is much more than that – to you, she is a partner, a friend and a confidante; to others, she is a daughter, sister and mother. She was not put on this planet for the sole purpose of making your sandwiches and folding your laundry, nor should she be treated as such. Here are a few helpful hints to keep in mind when striving for the perfect relationship:

- Maintain open lines of communication, both so you can express yourself and so you can hear where she is coming from.

- Take time to treat her concerns with the same consideration you treat your own; after all, any problem of hers is a problem of yours, as well. Even if you don't have any solutions, simply being supportive can go a long way.

- Identify her quirks and learn to love them as best you can. Hopefully she will be doing the same for you. A lot of the time it's those little things that make us who we are, so they should be appreciated.

- Be patient. Remember, the two of you aren't prisoners on a chain gang. For whatever reason you chose one another, you should remember that you are allies, not antagonists. Even during moments of conflict this remains true, as anyone who remains adamant about proving themselves right and "winning" will inevitably come out as a loser.

- Foreplay starts in the morning and continues throughout the day.

This last one is particularly important, as it is a grand part of what separates romantic relationships from other sorts of interaction. It is true, we all have needs (in fact, we have spent the last few chapters making quite sure of that), and that includes your significant other. Rather than view this is as some sort of burden, it should be undertaken as a collaborative effort. By staying in tune with one another, it is entirely possible to remain conscious and attentive to the other's physical desires.

It doesn't always start and end in the bedroom, however, unless you mean strictly in terms of romance beginning the moment you wake up and ending when you go to sleep. Intimacy is as much a mental game as it is a physical one, and should be treated as such. Remember, if a woman isn't in the mood – it ain't happening! By taking the time to get to know your partner in every sense of the word, it is possible to fulfill her on levels inaccessible by sheer physicality. Consideration and thoughtfulness go a long way in this regard and, of course, a woman who feels truly cared for and respected will be all the more willing to engage in regular S-E-X.

Women's Supplements

While they are, in fact, our better halves, women are not entirely problem-free. They face some of the same battles as we do during the Beer Belly Blues, experiencing impaired health and bodily function along with the diminished sex-hormone production that comes with aging. Just as we looked at in the previous chapter devoted to alternative remedies for men, women can often overcome hormonal imbalance naturally and side-effect free. Here as some of the most popular nutrients for promoting female health:

Peruvian Maca – A multipurpose herbal supplement we've already discussed, maca is just as useful to the lady in your life as it is for you.

Its influence on the endocrine system helps it to balance estrogen levels, which becomes especially erratic in the menopausal years. Its other health benefits, such as helping to maintain cholesterol, carry over as well. Aside from these incredibly important areas, maca might just be one of the most powerful aphrodisiacs any woman can try, as one woman bluntly put it, "I had to go off of maca because I didn't have a man in my life." Nuff said!

Indole-3-Carbinol – Yet another repeat from the natural supplements chapter, I3C is an extremely powerful antioxidant that is integral in maintaining appropriate estrogen levels. In fact, research appearing in the *Journal of Nutrition* noted that I3C has the ability to prevent the development of estrogen-enhanced cancers, including breast, endometrial and cervical cancers. It has also been tested as a treatment for diseases including lupus, which occurs almost nine times more frequently in women than it does in men, and human papillomavirus, a condition that leads to a high rate of cervical cancer.

Broccoli Extract – As broccoli is a cruciferous plant, it contains high levels of I3C. Additionally, it contains an element known as *sulforaphane*, which is being studied for its purported ability to prevent breast cancer by inhibiting the production of cancer stem cells. In lieu of effective chemotherapy, sulforaphane is thought to offer a reasonable alternative for treatment due to its ability to target and eradicate harmful cells, preventing tumor growth.

D-Glucarate – A naturally occurring substance found in fruits and vegetables, D-Glucarate has been shown to help in the removal of harmful materials such as toxins and carcinogens from the body. Studies have shown it to be especially useful in preventing breast cancer.

Holy Basil – In addition to being regarded by Hindus as a sacred avatar of the goddess Lakshmi, and a staple of Thai cuisine (though not to be confused with Thai basil or Thai lemon basil), holy basil is thought to have a number of health benefits, including reducing stress. Its levels of the active nutrient, *eugenol,* puts it on par with a number of prescription painkillers, and it has been studied for its potential as an anti-cancer agent. Its oil contains powerful antioxidant properties, an important consideration in maintaining healthy cholesterol levels.

Turmeric – Perhaps best known for its culinary applications, turmeric is also receiving a great deal of attention from the medical community as of late for the potential healing abilities of curcumin, one of its main components. With a historic use dating back over a thousand years in the Indian Ayurvedic medical tradition, curcumin is now being investigated by modern researchers as a treatment for conditions as diverse as pancreatitis, various forms of cancer and herpes.

Milk Thistle Extract – For years venerated as a "liver tonic," it is easy to see how milk thistle extract might encourage the healthy production of sex hormones. In addition to its effects on the liver, including helping to prevent cirrhosis and repairing damage caused by long-term exposure to toxins (such as alcohol or chemotherapy), milk thistle is also thought to help lower cholesterol and to inhibit the growth of cancer cells.

Oxytocin – the Love Hormone

No chapter honoring the women in our lives would be complete without a shoutout to one of the most important hormones a woman can experience, *oxytocin* – the Love Hormone. This is because it inspires a feeling of closeness, bonding and, yes, love. Often it is the hormone that is linked to childbirth and nurturing, but it has much greater implications than that. Of course it does. Why else would I waste critical Beer Belly Blues learning time on something that, save some strange and not necessarily welcome scientific advancements, we will never have to deal with?

Ah, have we forgotten so quickly the impact babies have on our testosterone? If you really want to boost your testosterone, stave off that beer belly and enjoy great quality of life, you have to appreciate the woman in your life – and that means learning about what makes her tick. I've already talked about some of the supplements that can help her feel her best, but now I'm going to delve into the highly-important hormone oxytocin and what it means to her.

Babies, Babies Everywhere, and Not a Drop to Spare

One of the most important functions of oxytocin is the benefit it provides women during labor, childbirth and postpartum periods. This hormone provides the physiological benefit of helping the cervix to soften and dilate, and the uterus to contract. All of this makes it much easier for the baby to see his/her new world. Another important function of oxytocin during labor is the calm, peaceful feelings and pain reduction that it offers. It's kind of natures epidural. In the very last moments of birth the woman's body will release a strong dose of the hormone. This encourages her body to push the baby out, while helping her to endure the strain.

What does this mean for you? Well, if your partner is one of the super-women that decide to refuse any pain medication during labor and birth, this little hormone can do wonders in saving the bones in your hand from being pulverized during each contraction. Oxytocin provides a feeling of well-being, and helps to manage the pain of labor so that the woman can keep working toward the actual delivery. You want your laboring partner to have nice high levels of oxytocin.

After birth, oxytocin goes to work bringing about all of those warm and fuzzy new mommy feelings. As soon as she touches the new baby, especially if there is skin-to-skin contact, she will get flooded with the hormone. This will make her love the baby and want to care for it – and possibly maul anyone who gets too close to her cub. It will also get the milk factory pumping. You may have noticed that she has been kind of leaky during the last couple of months of pregnancy, which is the forerunner of her making the milk to feed the baby. Once that oxytocin hits, though, her body will become a full-blown baby bar. Each time the new little one goes for one of her nipples, her brain will get the order and send the milk on down.

An intriguing study has also suggested that high levels of oxytocin, particularly those that are released after a positive social interaction or pleasant experience (such as meeting that adorable squishy newborn), can improve wound healing by reducing inflammation. For a woman that has just given birth, healing is a very important concept.

Pre-Baby Love Hormone

So now you know what oxytocin does for a childbearing woman. But what does it do for your partner *before* the baby – hopefully, in order to *get* the baby? Much like during birth, oxytocin creates feelings of emotional connection and love. This is scientifically referred to as the "ooey-gooey" effect. All right, not scientifically, but it does sound good. Studies have indicated that these feelings of affection and connection are particularly strong during sexual arousal and after orgasm. So all of those times when the school counselor said "sex doesn't equal love" didn't appreciate the effect of oxytocin on a woman's brain.

This bond doesn't just last through the few minutes of cuddling (which are highly recommended if you want to keep your mate happy), but actually creates a lingering sense of security and trust with each other. That means that if you keep your woman's oxytocin flowing, she will feel protected, safe, calm and in control when she is near you. Of course this helps when you are trying to bring her to that big moment, but more importantly, it will boost that "My big strong man!" sensation that will make you feel like a super hero. All you need is a long shiny cape with a big "O" stitched on the back.

It isn't just the loving bond that is facilitated by the release of oxytocin during sex. Some studies have shown that, much like the uterus during labor, the muscles being used during orgasm will also contract specifically for the purpose of propelling your little swimmers toward the Promised Land.

Tips for Boosting Her Oxytocin

Now that you know how important oxytocin is to your partner's quality of life – and yours – don't you want to know how you can help her keep the Love Hormone flowing? Fortunately, I have some tips for you. Haven't I always promised to help you out?

Remember that I mentioned foreplay starting in the morning and going all day? Part of this is finding ways to show your partner physical affection throughout the day. Things like holding hands, kissing her cheek, walking with your arms around each other and cuddling will release the hormone and keep it at a consistently high level.

Encourage her to pet the cat. No, really, that wasn't a horribly inappropriate euphemism. Studies into the effect of pet ownership on a person's psychological well-being have indicated that spending some time with a beloved animal can have much the same oxytocin-boosting effect as cuddling with you – just without the heroic adoration afterward.

Give her reason to think of you when you are away. Again, not an uncomfortable turn of phrase. When a woman loves someone, each time she thinks of her partner there is an increase in her oxytocin. This means that you can ensure periodic hormone boosts throughout the day with simple gestures such as slipping a handwritten note into her lunch, sending her flowers at work, calling her unexpectedly, or stopping by to visit her. Anything that will give her reason to think of you and smile.

I saved the best for last: have lots of sex. You like that suggestion, don't you? We've spent so much of this book talking about your testosterone and how to keep the fire burning, now I'm telling you that it's not just for your benefit. You want to keep up your sex drive for *her*. Women who have satisfying sex lives with their partners have consistently higher oxytocin levels. So go ahead and take one for the team.

Summary

What a long, strange trip it's been, right? It seems like just minutes ago you were opening the front cover, perhaps a bit curious as to what this whole testosterone deal is about, and then – BAM! – here you are, two-thirds of the way through your education in Beer Belly Blues-ology. If you need to take a breather, that's totally fine. I understand. Refresh your beverage, pop a new bowl of popcorn (with any of the diet-friendly oils suggested earlier, of course), and fluff your pillow, because we've got more ground to cover. But until the testosterone train leaves the station, let's review some of the information covered in the last section.

In **Section I** we took a basic look at testosterone and the role it plays in a number of basic bodily systems. We learned that our foe, the Beer Belly Blues, is like the ultimate guerilla warfare soldier. You can be going along, minding your own business, and it suddenly jumps out at you. Then once you learn to cope with that, it sneaks up on you again, but in a completely different part of your body. I told you about testosterone's critical impact on your heart, your brain, your prostate, your muscles, your energy and, yes, your unit. This was a foundation for our real mission as the Beer Belly Blues army. In **Section II** we got a little more in depth with the science in reference to the hows and the whys of the way things work.

Though we've seen the word "testosterone" about a thousand times so far, it is important to remember that it doesn't always mean the same thing. In terms of biochemistry, we learned that not all testosterone is created equal, and why total testosterone levels are not as important to understanding the true story of our hormone status as is the quantity of free (unbound) testosterone. Because testosterone is only one of many sex hormones seemingly running rampant through your body, we also touched on other hormones and how they work to strengthen your fight against the Beer Belly Blues. We discussed the role played by sex hormone binding globulin (SHBG) in affecting testosterone levels, as they tie up the most important form of testosterone – the free bioavailable testosterone – and thereby compromise its value. We also talked about the dangers posed by inflated aromatase levels, particularly in creating an overabundance of estrogen in the form of estradiol as we age. Though it might have inspired you to start comparing beige and ivory bras (not to mention the black lacey ones, of course) to see which looks best with your skin tone, I promised that I would give you a way to stave off any unwanted growth. I am a man of my word – only a little more patience, please!

We moved on to talk about how important nutrition is in both supporting and boosting your testosterone levels and in keeping your body and mind strong – even when facing down the Beer Belly Blues. In terms of nutrition, we reveled that not all cholesterol is evil and, is, in fact, absolutely fundamental to the production of testosterone. By maintaining a high ratio of HDL to LDL, one can not only ensure their health, but also avoid the considerable risks associated with taking the statins prescribed for mismanaged cholesterol. Though I didn't directly encourage a dance of celebration dedicated to egg salad, I was tempted. Cholesterol is one of the most misunderstood nutrients, and it really should be given some respect! We also took a look at the dual pillars of the human diet, fat and protein, both in terms of how they function and the benefits they offer. Also pretty misunderstood, I told you all of the ways that fat and protein come together to help your body to function correctly into middle age and beyond.

Beyond food, we investigated a few popular natural supplements that can be used to both bolster the effects of a well-planned diet and render synthetic substances such as ED drugs irrelevant. This is important because we are part of a society that has become far too dependent on pharmaceuticals to take care of issues that can be thoroughly and effectively approached using natural substances and lifestyle changes. Not only are drugs often less effective than these measures, but they can actually be dangerous. And be honest, do you really want something deemed potentially harmful and injurious near your erection? Probably not. Stay strong, Beer Belly Army, you are almost at the point where I'll tell you how to take charge and change your life without ever having to talk to a pharmacist or receive a plain paper package on your front porch.

After that, we evaluated some important lifestyle choices. Though I talked a bit in the first section about how reduced activity during middle age is a major contributing factor to the development of the beer belly, saggy muscles, reduced heart health and overall dip in testosterone (that, as we all know, just makes all of those things worse all over again), it is important to go into more detail about what exercise really is, and what it does for our bodies. That's why I told you that physical activity, while always an important part of one's health maintenance routine, is especially effective and approachable when conducted via the Biocize method. This method maximizes your efforts and lets you take full advantage of the time and energy that you have to dedicate to your physical activity. Furthermore, we took a moment to recognize our better halves and how important they truly are in our efforts to construct the ideal life. You might not have expected to read much about her in a book about decreased testosterone, but she has just too much impact to overlook. And yes, a great relationship is also very supportive of a healthy testosterone status.

It sure seems like we have covered a lot of ground, and that's with good reason: we have! I know it seems like an awful lot to remember (hence this handy cheat sheet), but it all fits together perfectly with a little bit of planning and a whole lot of practice. In the next section, we will review a few plans that show how easy it is to integrate all of this knowledge into a single comprehensive program to make sure that its the best version of you possible taking on the Beer Belly Blues. Are you ready, Beer Belly Blues Army? Fall into formation, because here we go!

Part III

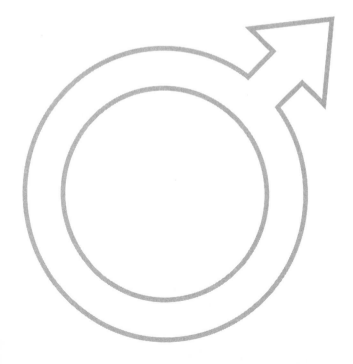

Putting It All Together

Well, we are finally near the end of our journey. Actually, as clichéd as it may sound, I would much rather you think of this as the beginning of the rest of your life ... lest we forget that you're about to become the Ultimate Male! In Part III you're going to learn how to take all that newfound knowledge in your noggin and put it to work for you.

In order to help you achieve whatever your health goals are, I'm going to start by sharing with you my top 10 tips for successfully navigating the Beer Belly Blues battlefield.

And to guide you on your journey, I am going to show you exactly how to eat – with a seven-day example of Ultimate Male easy-to-prepare delicious recipes even a non-chef like myself can make – seriously. You're also going to learn how to supplement the Ultimate Male way. I've even broken your supplement program into three easy-to-follow protocols depending on how serious you are ready to be with your Ultimate Male program. And in order to leave little-to-no room for failure, there's even a chapter on what to do to make your Biocize program as effective as possible.

Finally, you will learn what a real male-hormone panel should consist of, and what your blood levels of each of the hormones should be in order to emulate you at your peak of health and vitality. Yes, you're going to feel like a twenty-year-old again – let's just hope you don't act like one! And if you do, as the disclaimer at the front of the book says, "Not my problemo!"

Ok, Mr. Manly Man, enough with the wait-for-the-perfect day attitude – after all, when does that perfect day ever come anyway?. Let's get started, shall we?

Chapter Twenty One:
The Top 10 Beer Belly Blues Banishers

1) Change Your Attitude

According to myriad studies, your mind and attitude may be one of the most important factors when it comes to impacting testosterone in a positive manner. In other words, you will need to swap out the constant negative beliefs and self-talk for more positive ones (as one has-been sitcom star recently ranted over and over again, WINNING!). Well, testosterone loves a winning attitude, whereas a losing one causes testosterone levels to plummet. Researchers from Syracuse University in New York discovered that testosterone levels rise right before a challenge, as if testosterone automatically increases when men face competition. The researchers also found that once the competition is over, testosterone levels rise in winners and decline in losers. However, it is of utmost importance for a man to boost his mood before experiencing an increase in testosterone, so get that winning attitude in motion.

To further support the science that a healthy attitude is the enemy of the Beer Belly Blues, research also shows that replacing negative emotions with positive ones is a clear way to healthier testosterone levels. A study performed at the Institute of HeartMath in Boulder Creek, California, used techniques that were designed to eliminate negative thought patterns and promote a positive emotional state. The 30 subjects in the study showed a 23-percent reduction in the body's premiere stress hormone, cortisol (cortisol competes with testosterone), and a 100-percent increase in DHEA/DHEA-S levels, which are often correlated with testosterone levels.

Action: Well, change your attitude and become that positive person you've always wanted to be. Try baby steps like actually smiling more and immediately correcting a negative action by exchanging it with a positive one.

2) Stress Less

When we constantly stress over things, we end up elevating our stress hormones – especially cortisol. Perception equals reality in the face of stress. During stress, cortisol can easily become more important to your body than other hormones, and since it is produced along the same biochemical pathway as your sex hormones, it usually ends robbing the body of the very substances needed to keep these hormones in abundance.

One of the reasons our libidos are almost non-existent during times of stress is that cortisol often competes with testosterone. If this wasn't bad enough, cortisol also competes with dehydroepiandrosterone (DHEA), your anti-aging hormone, which is why people seem to magically age before your eyes when they are under stress for long periods. DHEA is also needed to maintain a healthy metabolism.

In normal metabolisms, there is a balance between testosterone and cortisol, which creates a healthy balance between the body's breakdown (cortisol/catabolism) and repair (testosterone/anabolism) processes. Stress tips the odds in favor of breakdown, and thus the body has a harder and harder time keeping up with the damage. Premature aging is exactly this process – the body's inability to repair faster than the damage occurs. By upsetting the natural process of breakdown and repair, stress, in turn, makes us fat because it also contributes to insulin resistance. This invariably puts our body into a fat-storage mode (due to the need for excess insulin) and greatly increases our risk of the metabolic syndrome, which you already know completely obliterates your testosterone levels.

Action: Do whatever you can to reduce stress in your life. This usually starts with making a conscious effort not to overreact to little things within your life and to start breathing deeper. You can also try *Peruvian Maca,* or research-proven Anti-Stress or Ultimate Calm formulas that contain ingredients such as *GABA* (in the form of PharmaGABA), *Ashwagandha, Rhodiola* and *Valerian.*

3) Lose the Grump

Now at first glance you would think that that a bad attitude and a low mood may be one in the same. They are not! Low mood, or depression, is a serious issue that affects millions of North Americans, so much so that according to my friend and colleague, Dr. Michael Murray, more than 10 percent of the North American population is now on drugs that are supposedly designed to combat depression. The worst part of all is that approximately three-quarters of these people don't experience any results from these drugs.

In terms of your precious testosterone, if you want to banish the Beer Belly Blues you absolutely have to eliminate depression from your life. In fact, according to studies, men with abnormally low testosterone are, on average, **271 percent** more likely to show clinical signs of depression than men with higher testosterone levels.

Another way in which depression causes testosterone levels to plummet is by elevating stress hormones (primarily cortisol). Actually, cortisol itself may be a cause of depression. It comes down to which came first, the chicken or the egg. According to Harvard-trained neurologist, Dr. Jeff Victoroffe, approximately 50 percent of people who suffer from severe depression also have elevated cortisol levels. The problem is that cortisol happens to be a major destroyer of brain cells – primarily the hippocampal neurons associated with both short-term and long-term memory – ultimately leading to further depression. If this wasn't enough, there is also a strong link between depression and erectile dysfunction, which is depressing enough in its own right.

Action: If you suffer from depression, get a medical diagnosis as soon as possible. Do your research on the numerous prescription meds for depression before taking any, as there are numerous natural alternatives available without side effects, such as suicide!

4) Sleep Better

Deep restorative sleep is one of the best ways to ensure healthy testosterone levels. Testosterone levels ebb and flow throughout the day and night, usually peaking in the early morning and declining from there (8 P.M. is usually when testosterone levels are at their lowest). Deep sleep (referred to as phases III and IV) enhances your body's ability to produce testosterone. According to studies, the deeper and more uninterrupted your sleep patterns, the more testosterone can be produced (within reason, of course). In fact, researchers from the University of Chicago discovered that sleep quality was greatest independent predictor of testosterone levels (both free and total) in older men.

The main problem is that men actually lose the ability to get into deeper sleep cycles as they age and lose testosterone, so it becomes an ever-increasing double-edged sword. Researchers from the University of Montreal in Canada recently discovered that the decline in testosterone levels most men experience with age was to blame for much of these sleep problems. Younger men typically spend 10-20 percent of their total sleep in deep-sleep phases, whereas most 50 year olds are lucky to experience 5-6 percent deep-sleep phases. By the time men are 60, deep-sleep phases are almost nonexistent.

Action: Aim for at least 8 hours of sleep each night, and try to go to bed before 10 P.M. for best effects. If you need a sleep aid, do not use prescription meds, as they have little to no effect on deep sleep, and come with numerous side effects. Instead try natural ingredients like; *tryptophan, 5-HTP, lysine, melatonin, L Theanine* and *Jujube (zizyphus spinosa) fruit.*

5) Find Your Mojo

I know you probably already know this, but just in case you don't, here it is: "Sex is great!" Of course it is. However I am referring to the way a healthy sex life helps support your testosterone levels. Sex has been known to support and enhance testosterone for years. A study at Georgia State University in Atlanta, suggests that testosterone levels rise after sexual activity. The study reviewed couples before and after sexual intercourse on a total of 11 evenings followed by 11 evenings with no intercourse. It turns out that testosterone increased – in both men and women – across the entire evening when there was intercourse, but decreased when there was none. Other studies suggest that even the thought of having sex helps to increase testosterone. No wonder we pumped out so much of the stuff in our teens and twenties!

On the other side of the coin, when a man experiences the Beer Belly Blues, one of the first things to go is sexual desire (a.k.a your libido), often followed by the inability to experience or keep a healthy erection (a.k.a: our old friend ED). Studies indicate that men who suffer from ED usually experience lower testosterone levels due to a lack of sex.

Action: If you are someone who has low libido, ED or both, you may want to try natural libido-enhancing nutritionals such as the ones mentioned in **Chapter Eighteen: Ultimate Male Supplements.**

6) Say No to Sugar

Sugar is a fancy word for carbohydrates and excess carbohydrates (not including fibrous vegetables) create a fat-storage environment within the body – primarily around the abdominal cavity – by stimulating high insulin levels. One of insulin's primary jobs in the body is to store fat for future use. However, it also prevents the body from getting at that fat, further exacerbating obesity. As the beer belly expands, so do its estrogen-manufacturing abilities, because the enzyme that converts testosterone into estrogen lives within the subcutaneous layer of belly fat. Thus, excess sugar (carbohydrate) = more insulin = more abdominal-fat storage = more aromatase = more estrogen and less testosterone.

Aside from insulin's role (no pun intended) in expanding your fat cells, after meal (post prandial) blood-sugar spikes have also been shown to lead to decreased testosterone levels – by a whopping 25 percent! The problem is that most North Americans already experience excessively high blood sugar levels – especially after a carbohydrate-rich meal. Nutritional researchers have now come to the conclusion that a healthy blood sugar level should be 85 mg/dL or less, and numerous problems – including obesity, cardiovascular disease, cancer, cataracts, prostate disease, liver damage, sleep apnea and low testosterone – increase exponentially when blood sugar levels are sustained above this level.

In order to help reduce excess blood sugar levels, first of all do your best to avoid high-glycemic carbohydrates – primarily grains and potatoes – especially during the last meal of the day (follow the guidelines in the Ultimate Male Solutions Meal Guidelines and Seven Days of Recipes in this section).

Action: Try supplementing with research-proven nutrients that can help lower post-meal blood-sugar spikes, such as *organic fiber*, *chlorogenic acid*, *cinnamon extract*, *green-tea extract*, *Phaseolamin* or *Phase 2™* and *Gymnema Sylvestre*.

7) Get Some Sun

I remember not so long ago when lying in the sun was not such a bad thing. I'm not referring to exposing yourself to the strongest sunlight in order to burn, but merely exposing your skin to the sun long enough to produce one of the most vital compounds that we have ever discovered – vitamin D. Vitamin D is far from just another essential vitamin. In fact, it really isn't a vitamin at all, due to the fact that it functions as a type of hormone (*prohormone*), and because the body can make it (as vitamin D_3) as long as there is adequate sun exposure. The main problem is that nowadays everyone uses sunscreen and is afraid to go out in the sun for fear of getting skin cancer. Unfortunately this is just not true. A lack of sunshine on your skin may be a *much larger cause* of many cancers than lying in the sun ever was! In fact, my colleague, Dr. Loren Cordain, author of the bestseller, *The Paleo Diet,* and professor in the Health and Exercise Science Department at Colorado State University, writes in his new book, *The Paleo Answer*, "Chronic, long-term exposure to the sun, such as what lifeguards and other outdoor workers experience, is protective from melanomas and many other cancers, whereas intermittent, infrequent, intense burning followed by little sun exposure, may promote the deadly form of skin cancer and many other cancers."

Regardless of vitamin D's skin-protective abilities, it turns out that the sunshine vitamin also has the ability to positively influence testosterone levels. Austrian researcher's recently discovered that men who have the lowest levels of vitamin D also have the lowest levels of testosterone. The researchers also pointed out that those men with the highest levels of vitamin D experience higher levels of testosterone. So, if you want to support optimal testosterone levels it may be wise to supplement with vitamin D.

Action: Try exposing your skin to direct sunlight – but avoid burning – in the early morning or late afternoon for 10-15 minutes. When or if you are unable to do this, try supplementing with at least **2,000 units** of vitamin D3. However, the Life Extension Foundation has analyzed more than 13,000 vitamin-D blood tests, which led them to announce that the minimum intake for most aging people should be around **7,000 IU a day**. If you get your personal vitamin-D levels checked (referred to as 25-Hydroxy Vitamin D), aim for a blood level of approximately **50 ng/mL**.

8) Lose the Belly

As mentioned throughout this book, belly fat is a manufacturing plant for estrogen by virtue of it becoming a prime location for the aromatase enzyme. Men become so efficient at producing estrogen (estradiol) from testosterone that many can easily become estrogen dominant.

In fact, estrogen levels are so closely linked to excess belly fat that a large waist circumference – 100 cm (40 inches) or more – can often be a determining factor of low testosterone and high estrogen levels. As you read in the estrogen chapter, high estrogen is often responsible for abdominal obesity, loss of energy, low moods, heart disease, diabetes, cancer, prostate disease, and the dreaded man-boob syndrome.

Another reason to do everything in your power to lose the beer belly is that excess abdominal fat is linked to diabetes and the metabolic syndrome, and these conditions are associated with lower testosterone levels and higher morbidity and mortality rates. In fact, a study appearing in the *Journal of Men's Health* indicated that low testosterone might actually be a major contributing factor to the metabolic syndrome. Aside from this, it is well documented that men who are obese produce less testosterone then men who are of normal weight.

Action: Lose the belly by following the guidelines in Part III of this book.

9) Don't Overtrain

This one won't apply to the majority of men, as most do not exactly enjoy working out. However, if you are anything like me, you love to train – whether it be hitting the weights or going for an uphill run in the woods – sometimes too much! You already know from reading Chapter Nineteen on Biocize that high-impact exercise is great for enhancing anabolic (rebuild and repair) hormones such as testosterone, but too much of a good thing can have just the opposite effect –whacking testosterone into the ground.

Numerous studies show that overtraining can lead to a precipitous decline in testosterone, sometimes for days afterward. So it becomes imperative to listen to your body and respect it when it tells you to take a break. This becomes ever more important with advanced age, as the body is less able to recuperate as quickly as it did when you were younger. To make matters worse, numerous studies show that overtraining leads to a compromised immune system, opening the door to opportunistic viral and bacterial infections, which further close the door on healthy testosterone production.

Action: If you are experiencing excessive soreness, low energy, depressed moods or frequent bouts of illness (i.e. colds or flue like symptoms), it's time to reevaluate how often or hard you are training and take a much-needed break. Also, read Tip #10 (Up Your BCAAs), as BCAAs are a great way to help reduce or overcome the overtraining syndrome.

10) Up Your BCAAs

As I detailed in Chapter Seventeen, BCAAs are a group of three essential amino acids (leucine, isoleucine and valine) that are extremely beneficial when it comes to fat loss and supporting your body's regenerative ability. Studies also indicate they are very important when it comes to supporting healthy testosterone levels.

Researchers from Ball State University found that BCAAs have the ability to exert powerful effects by altering testosterone and cortisol in a favorable fashion. The study involved a group of bodybuilders who were given 6 grams of BCAAs daily over a four-week period. For the first three weeks, the bodybuilders took the supplement without exercise, but the fourth week they performed high-intensity total-body resistance exercise along with taking the supplements. With just one week of combined exercise and BCAA supplementation, testosterone levels rose almost 50 percent above baseline. If this wasn't enough proof, BCAA supplementation significantly reduced muscle damage from the workouts.

Action: Try supplementing with a *High-Alpha Whey Protein Isolate* (which contains almost seven grams of BCAAs per serving), *BCAA capsules*, or add the amino acid *leucine* (the king of the BCAAs) to your existing protein shake).

Chapter Twenty Two:

Ultimate Male Solutions Eating Principles

It's Time to Lose the Belly. I have never known anyone to get excited about starting a diet, which is exactly why it is so important for men to learn what to eat and how to eat. It's about embracing the proper foods at the proper times of the day – NOT ABOUT COUNTING CALORIES! That's right, I am not a believer in calorie counting for the very reason that this method of fat loss is very rarely, if ever, successful – especially in the long term. Also, it is not recommended for men who are interested in maintaining a healthy testosterone status.

You'll notice I used the term "fat loss" as opposed to "weight loss." This is because caloric deprivation-type diets do nothing to ensure that you will hold onto valuable muscle tissue, which is essential if your goal is to become the Ultimate Male. In fact, very often fad diets (i.e. low-calorie or low-fat diets) cause you to lose just as much muscle as fat, which is not smart if you truly want to lose the belly and all the estrogen that comes along with it.

This section contains real strategies that have been proven to work on real people. It's not in any way a fad diet, but a program you can follow for life. Aside from all this, who wants to count every calorie every day for the rest of their lives anyway?

The reason I am so convinced that the principles outlined in this section will help you lose the belly and gain the testosterone edge, is because these very principles have been used – with much success – for over ten years by tens of thousands of people all over the world. My first book, *Fat Wars: 45 Days to Transform Your Body*, changed thousands of people's lives for the better. The science of fat loss is my first love (aside from my family, of course), and nothing brings me greater pleasure than to see people who follow my protocols become successful – even when countless other programs have failed them.

Eat, Enjoy, Embrace

The Ultimate Male Solution eating principles are based upon portion control for your individual uniqueness. After following the eating plan for a relatively short period of time, your body will adjust its metabolism to allow its own fat stores to become the preferred source of fuel for your body.

It is important to note that **The Ultimate Male Solution** eating principles are about *eating*, *enjoying* and *embracing* nutrient-dense foods rather than *avoiding* them. Now there's a concept you can sink your teeth into! It is also important to understand that this section is designed to educate you on how to eat to achieve and maintain a healthy metabolism with enough testosterone for the rest of your life. This in no way means that you can never reward yourself with so-called "fun foods" (and you know what these are), but the goal is to establish a healthy metabolism with optimal testosterone levels first (which can take a few months) before you start including "fun foods" in your diet.

The Ultimate Male Solution eating principles consist of consuming proper nutrition (including effective supplementation) at regular intervals throughout the day. This is why I advocate eating three solid meals and consuming two high-quality protein shakes – preferable from High-Alpha Whey Protein – per day. For optimal metabolic effect these meals are to be consumed every three to four hours. By consuming smaller portions of nutrient-dense foods throughout the day, your body is able to balance blood sugar chemistry, keep insulin levels in check, support proper hormone chemistry, and reduce cravings more effectively.

To function optimally, the human body requires essential nutrients – nutrients that your body cannot manufacture on its own. These are: **water**, **minerals**, **vitamins**, **carbohydrates**, **fats** and **proteins**.

Water regulates all functions of the body.

Minerals regulate processes within the body that help generate enzymes, hormones, skeletal bones, muscle, teeth and fluids (visit **www. LeafSource.com** for one of the best natural organic trace-mineral formulas available today).

Vitamins are found in fruits, vegetables, meats and whole grains. Vitamins provide energy to the body and are needed in small amounts to assist the chemical reactions within our cells.

Proteins help stabilize blood sugar, promote cell growth and repair, assist hormone production and enzyme production (digestive and metabolic), as well as neurotransmitter production, cell metabolism, body-fluid balancing, maintenance of the immune system, and are essential to healthy testosterone levels (see Chapter Seventeen).

Carbohydrates (only the low glycemic/non-processed variety) ensure energy production, thyroid conversion and muscular repair, and help maintain a proper balance of insulin to glucagon to ensure effective fat burning.

Fats (as in essential fatty acids – EFA's, good saturated fats (think coconut oil and egg yolks, and monounsaturated fats) – are essential to produce energy, construct cellular membranes, help detoxify the body, regulate cell traffic (keeping viruses and germs out, and cell proteins, organelles, enzymes and genetic material in), maintain healthy insulin functions, form red blood cells, lubricate our joints, and help us maintain an optimal metabolism. Good fats also ensure that we burn fat by increasing the amount of oxygen utilized by the cells to produce energy, and they are essential to healthy testosterone levels (see Chapter Sixteen).

Constructing Your Ultimate Male Meals

When planning an **Ultimate Male** friendly meal, it is important to include all essential nutrients. We all know how to find water, but what about the rest of these nutrients? Your vitamins and minerals should come primarily from fruits and vegetables (and supplementation is also wise – see chapter Twenty-Three); however, it is important to note that conventionally grown foods can contain up to 90 percent fewer minerals than their organic counterparts.

The following is a quick overview as to which foods are **Ultimate Male** friendly, and fall under the categories of **protein**, **carbohydrates** and **fats**.

Ultimate Male Proteins:

- **Fish** – salmon, cod, tuna, bass, halibut, snapper, swordfish, trout, haddock and sole.

- **Seafood** – shrimp, scallops, lobster, crab, clams, oysters and mussels.

- **Poultry** – free range: chicken breast, turkey breast, duck, ostrich, goose and quail.

- **Meat** – game meats and tenderloin.

- **Eggs** – organic and free run (cage free).

- **Milk products** (although I am not a big proponent of milk and it's many byproducts, if you do decide to consume milk products try to stick to these choices) – plain organic yogurt (goat is the best) and cottage cheese.

- **Protein formulas** – whey protein (preferably High-Alpha Whey Protein), hemp, sprouted brown rice and Sacha inchi.

Ultimate Male Carbohydrates:

Fruits (preferably berries), vegetables (all non-starchy – think lots of green leafy ones), nuts and legumes.

Ultimate Male Healthy Fats:

Egg yolks, olive oil, avocados, almonds, walnuts, fish oil, hempseed (and its oil), flax (and its oil), pumpkin seeds, Brazil nuts, krill, sunflowers, cashews and pistachio nuts.

The Best Fats and Oils for Cooking

- Olive Oil (extra virgin-cold pressed)
- Coconut Oil
- Walnut Oil
- Avocado Oil
- Butter

(when cooking with these oils, cook over low to medium temperatures only)

Measuring Your Protein Portion

When it comes to constructing a properly designed **Ultimate Male** meal, you should always start by fulfilling your protein needs. To do this, your protein choice should be the approximate *size* and *thickness of your palm*, which should equate to approximately **4-6oz.**

Healthy Eggs

I recommend free-range, organic omega-3 eggs for a couple of reasons. Free-range chickens are just that – free to roam and feed off the land as chickens were intended to do – and happy chickens usually equate to healthy chickens. As well, when chickens are raised on feed that is fortified with omega-3 fats, their eggs contain elevated levels of these beneficial fats, which, as you will recall, are not as abundant in our diet as their omega-6 counterparts.

Adding Your Carbohydrates and Healthy-Fat Portions

Once you have your selected choice of protein, fill the rest of your plate with fibrous vegetables (which come from the recommended carbohydrate choices). Now this does not mean that you have to have salad every single night. Your vegetables can be steamed, broiled, baked or poached.

For the healthy fat portion of your **Ultimate Male** meals, use the healthy fat recommendations as salad dressings or vegetable toppings (such as seeds and nuts).

Nuts and Seeds

All nuts and seeds must be fresh, unsalted, un-roasted and blanched (if the nut has a skin). Raw is your best bet.

- Almonds .... 10 (average serving)
- Cashews .... 9 (average serving)
- Pecans .... 8 (average serving)
- Pumpkin seeds .... 20 (average serving)
- Pistachios .... 22 (average serving)
- Walnuts .... 7 (average serving)
- Sunflower seeds .... 25 (average serving)

Organic Is Always Best

Given an option, organic is always your best bet. Organic foods supply an enhanced nutritional value to your body's structure, and are similar to the foods our ancestors ate. Organic foods are also free from unnecessary chemicals, preservatives, contaminants, and other harmful substances such as pesticides, herbicides and fungicides. According to the *Journal of Applied Nutrition*, the majority of organic fruits, vegetables and grains have 90 percent more minerals than conventionally grown food.

The Problem with Grains

When it comes to grains, it is important to note that many grains cause a rapid rise in your insulin response, which places your body in a fat-storing mode by elevating insulin and a powerful fat-storage enzyme called *lipoprotein lipase* or LPL. Aside from this, many people have a difficult time digesting gluten, which is the protein found in grains.

According to the book *Dangerous Grains*, gluten intolerance does not just affect people with Celiac Disease (CD) – an allergic reaction to the grain found primarily in rye, oats and barley – but a great percentage of our population. In fact, the authors suggest that CD should actually be renamed "gluten sensitivity." I have found that when men (and women) avoid all forms of grains – yes, even the so-called healthy ones – they look, feel and perform much better. The beautiful part about this reality is that most people notice benefits within the first few days or within a week.

Sweeteners

There are many different artificial sweeteners on the market, and it is in your best interest to familiarize yourself with the pros and cons of each. I am not a proponent of any artificial sweetener available today, as these were never around as our intricate biochemistry was evolving and therefore may present problems to our bodies. The only natural sweeteners I presently advocate are *Stevia* and *Xylitol*, as these are both 100-percent natural, and do not seem to negatively affect metabolism.

Beware of Fructose

Although fructose is considered a natural sugar (and it is in fruit), often when it is added to foods and beverages – especially as high-fructose corn syrup – it can greatly enhance our ability to store fat and decrease metabolism. According to the research of Richard Johnson, MD, chief of the division of kidney disease and hypertension at the University of Colorado and one of the world's leading experts in this area, excess fructose consumption can lead to high blood pressure, obesity and diabetes. Fruit juices contain exceptionally high levels of concentrated fructose – yes, even the "so-called" 100 percent natural juices. So beware!

Processed Foods

I highly recommend avoiding like the plague all processed foods! These foods do nothing but strip the body of its own nutrient supplies and, in the process, lower testosterone and elevate insulin levels, which ultimately make it next to impossible to use fat as energy.

Trans Fats

If you want to protect your valuable testosterone, I highly recommend avoiding foods containing trans fats. These fake fats have been found to raise levels of LDL cholesterol, which is a major cause of heart disease. Forty percent of daily trans fat intake among North Americans comes from cakes, cookies, crackers, pies, bread and the like.

Out On the Town

Looking for the keys to eating out and being sociable without blowing everything you worked so hard for? Your success at becoming the **Ultimate Male** is largely determined by your lifestyle and dietary choices. In fact, every time you sit down to eat you are either moving one step closer to a fat-burning metabolism – or one step closer to a fat-storing one. Each and every day, and perhaps each hour, you are in a position to make a choice that either advances your goals or sets them back.

Since it has taken most of us many years to transform into the shape and health we are presently experiencing, we cannot expect positive transformation overnight. One fat-promoting, testosterone-depleting meal can easily turn into a second and so on, just as one day of lethargy can turn into a second and so on. We all have choices. Unfortunately, too many of us take the easy road and end up breaking down long before we reach the end.

It is not always easy to make the right choices, but the bottom line is we all have to live with the choices we make. Some of the hardest choices come in the form of *what* and *when* to eat when we are out for dinner or out on the road. Far too often we make food choices unconsciously in an effort to satisfy a need that is not tangible at the time. We need to be preemptive and make sure we plan for behaviors and situations, so we are always one step ahead.

Part of a winning approach is to anticipate the situations that will trigger old behaviors of poor eating habits. To help you avoid defeating behaviors, I will provide you with scenarios that suggest how to stay on the **Ultimate Male Solution** road when eating out, during social situations and on the road.

Restaurant Eating

Despite our good intentions to make healthful meals, our lives are filled with competing interests that draw us to making convenient choices. When eating out at a restaurant, consider these strategies:

- When you have a choice, choose a restaurant that provides a varied menu. Stay away from menus that do not allow you to make healthy choices. Some examples include hamburger joints, fish-and-chip restaurants, fried-chicken outlets and barbecued-rib restaurants.

- While at the restaurant, be strategic and choose foods that are wholesome instead of processed. These unprocessed foods will not only provide you with the greatest amount of testosterone-supporting nutrients but also keep you full longer.

- Ask yourself questions when you are making a food choice at a restaurant. How much unhealthy fat does the food have? Does it contain good fats or bad ones? Fats provide the most calories for the lowest amount of nutrients. This is an important area to consider when you decide how much and what type of fat you will consume.

- When you sit down at a restaurant, sometimes a basket of bread gets brought to the table. It is always best to ask the waiter *not* to serve the bread at your table and avoid the temptation altogether. It is extremely rare to find a restaurant that serves healthier choices such as stone-ground or sprouted-grain breads, so it is best to **just say no**! Eating the bread will stimulate the fat-storing high-insulin response, add calories to your meal and provide you with very little nutrient density. If you are in a situation where others at your table want bread, do your very best to avoid eating it.

- Make sure you choose a main dish that is not starch-based. Choose meals that are high in protein and low in starchy carbohydrates. Most restaurants are very accommodating, so don't be afraid to ask your waiter for options.

- Make sure to include a good portion of fibrous mixed vegetables with your protein source. For instance, if you are ordering steak, chicken or fish, try to forgo the baked potato or rice pilaf and instead opt for a nice serving of veggies or a big salad.

Here are a few simple suggestions that will help you construct a healthier meal at any restaurant:

- Ask for dressings and sauces on the side – olive oil and vinaigrette are always the best option.

- Opt for fruit and/or vegetable-based sauces rather than creamy sauces.

- Choose meals that are poached, steamed, broiled or baked, but never fried.

- Say no to dessert, but if you can't, choose fruit or yogurt-based desserts. Have the occasional dark chocolate treat, but make that treat infrequent and small.

- Foods that contain more fibers tend to fill you up and control the release of your fat-storing hormone, insulin. Therefore:

- Avoid refined rice and any white-flour products, including pasta.

- Go for large amounts and a wide variety of vegetables. If necessary, ask for a larger portion of your favorite vegetables (or a big salad).

- Remember to ask for steamed, broiled, baked or poached vegetables that are not lathered in butter but lightly coated with olive oil.

Don't Be Fooled Again

Don't be fooled into the belief that beverages don't contain calories just because they don't contain fat. Alcoholic beverages can contain an enormous number of sugars and calories, and make you feel hungry rather than provide you with valuable nutrients. Always choose water as your beverage of choice at a restaurant and go for the glass of red wine once in a while. After all, you are human.

My Top 10 Ultimate Male Solution Eating Tips

- Consume five mini meals per day (three solid, and two protein shakes).

- Make sure to eat every three to four hours in order to maintain blood sugar levels.

- Include high-quality protein in each and every meal, making sure to individualize your protein portion (see **Measuring Your Protein Portion** in this chapter).

- Drink plenty of water. A good rule of thumb is to consume one liter of water for every 50 pounds of bodyweight, and don't forget to include 8 oz. of filtered water approximately 20 minutes prior to each meal in order to curb your appetite.

- Watch your consumption of fruit juices, as they often contain too much fructose, and completely avoid fruit drinks with added sugars.

- Don't be afraid of fat – just choose they healthy ones (see **Ultimate Male Healthy Fats** in this chapter).

- Never overeat.

- Eat slowly, and stop when you are no longer hungry.

- Don't consume carbs past 6:00 PM.

- Always leave at least two hours between your last meal and bedtime.

Top 10 Testosterone-Boosting Foods

- Oysters
- Game Meat (free run)
- Lean Beef (organic)
- Poultry (organic and/or free run)
- Eggs (organic and/or free run)
- Cottage Cheese (organic)
- Broccoli
- Cabbage
- Brussels Sprouts
- Garlic

The Ultimate Male Solution's Seven Days of Recipes

In this section you will find seven days' worth of testosterone-supporting recipes that are super easy to prepare. These recipes are constructed as three solid meals and two protein shakes/day for a total of 35 recipes in total. I want every man to see how simple and delicious it can be to adhere to a testosterone-supporting dietary protocol – one that will help you get back on track and become the Ultimate Male. You can choose to follow these recipes exactly or mix them up if you'd prefer. They are here to make your life a lot easier and with the guidelines listed above you will have no choice but to be successful on your journey, so BON APPETIT!

FIRST Meal of the Day Options:

Muesli

1 cup organic plain yogurt

2 tablespoons Muesli

1 scoop Strawberry High Alpha Whey Protein

½ small banana, sliced

¼ cup blueberries, fresh

In bowl, mix all ingredients together.

Egg no Muffin

2 eggs organic or free run, poached

2 tablespoons salsa

½ avocado

2 slices Peameal bacon or prosciutto, organic

Poach eggs to your liking. Cut up the avocado into bite-size pieces and mix with salsa. Place your poached eggs on top of your Peameal or prosciutto and cover with salsa mixture.

Fruit Salad with Cottage Cheese

1 cup cottage cheese

2 cups of fresh fruit of your liking. Recommended fruits include: berries, apples, grapefruit, oranges, nectarines, peaches, pear, plums or apricots.

2 tablespoons cashew pieces

Cut fruit into bite-size pieces; mix with cottage cheese and sprinkle cashews on top.

Spinach Omelet

3 eggs, organic or free run

¼ cup spinach

1 tablespoon feta cheese

2 slices red onion

1 tablespoon olive oil

2 teaspoons milk, organic

In a skillet, over medium heat, add ½ tablespoon olive oil, spinach and red onion. Sauté for 5 minutes. Remove from skillet. Add ½ tablespoon to skillet, pour in egg mixture (break eggs into bowl, add 2 teaspoons milk, and whisk) and cover with spinach, onion and feta cheese. Run spatula around skillet edge, and once the egg mixture is cooked on one side, flip one half of egg over on the other. Cook for a few minutes and then flip the omelet on its other side.

Granola yogurt

1 cup yogurt

⅓ cup granola (no sugar added)

½ cup berries

1 scoop vanilla High Alpha Whey Protein

1 tablespoon honey

Mix protein into yogurt, add granola and berries and drizzle with honey.

Quinoa Porridge

½ cup uncooked quinoa

1 cup water

½ teaspoon cinnamon

½ cup milk, organic

1 small Granny Smith apple, diced

½ cup blueberries

¼ cup walnuts, chopped

1 tablespoon maple syrup (optional)

In a small pot, place quinoa, water and cinnamon, and bring to a boil. Once boiling, reduce heat and cover on simmer for 15 minutes or until most of the water has been absorbed. Add milk and continue simmering uncovered for an additional 10 minutes. Stir in apple, blueberries and walnuts. Let sit covered for 10 minutes before serving. If you choose to add maple syrup, drizzle this on top.

Cheesy Egg Bake

2 eggs, lightly beaten

2 cups organic cottage cheese

¼ cup organic mozzarella, grated

2 green onions, chopped

Mix all ingredients together, and pour into oven-safe bake dish. Cook at 350 degrees for 45 to 50 minutes (depending on your oven). Let sit for a few minutes before serving.

SECOND Meal of the Day Options (liquid shakes):

Pina Colada

Strawberry Ultimate Protein .... 1 serving

Pineapple, tidbits or crushed .... ¼ cup

Coconut milk .... 1 tablespoon

In blender, mix pineapple and coconut milk with water. Blend well. Add Ultimate Protein and your chosen fat source for an additional 10 seconds on low.

Morning Maca Punch

Chocolate Ultimate Protein .... 1 serving

Ultimate Maca Punch .... 1 tablespoon

Almond milk .... 1 cup

Place Maca and almond milk in blender. Blend well. Add Ultimate Protein and your chosen fat source for an additional 10 seconds on low.

Detoxify and Feel Great!

Strawberry Ultimate Protein .... 1 serving

Lemon, freshly squeezed .... 1 tablespoon

Rhubarb .... ¼ cup

FibreLean .... ½ to 1 scoop

Place rhubarb, FibreLean and freshly squeezed lemon in blender with water. Blend well. Add Ultimate Protein and your chosen fat source for an additional 10 seconds on low.

Metabolism Booster Smoothie

Vanilla Ultimate Protein.. 1 serving

Raspberries.. ½ cup

Apple, small .... ¼

Core and skin apple. In blender, combine raspberries, apple and water. Blend well. Add Ultimate Protein and your chosen fat source for an additional 10 seconds on low.

Healthy Prostate Smoothie

Unflavored Ultimate Protein... 1 serving

Tomato juice, no sugar added.. 1 cup

Celery stalk 1

In blender, put tomato juice with celery. Blend well. Add Ultimate Protein and your chosen fat source for an additional 10 seconds on low.

Testosterone Booster

Vanilla Ultimate Protein.. 1 serving

Avocado .... ½

Kale.. ½ cup

In blender, blend avocado and kale using water as your medium. Blend well. Add Ultimate Protein and your chosen fat source for an additional 10 seconds on low.

Energy Shake

Strawberry Ultimate Protein .... 1 serving

Blackberries .... ¼ cup

Blueberries .... ¼ cup

Mango .... ¼ cup

Place berries, mango and water in blender. Blend well. Add Ultimate Protein and your chosen fat source for an additional 10 seconds on low.

THIRD Meal of the Day Options:

Lemon Chicken

1 organic or free range chicken breast

1 serving organic long whole grain rice

Organic chicken or vegetable broth (for cooking rice)

½ cup honey

2 tablespoons stone-ground mustard

1 tablespoon Dijon mustard

2 teaspoons curry

Cook rice according to instructions on bag or box. Cut chicken into slices. Mix honey, mustards and curry into a bowl. Add chicken and marinate for 15 minutes to 2 hours. Once rice is cooked, set aside. Over medium heat, cook chicken until done.

Just for the Halibut

1 serving Halibut

3 teaspoons olive oil

¼ cup diced zucchini

2 tablespoons onion. chopped finely

1 clove garlic, minced

¼ cup Roma tomatoes, chopped finely

1 tablespoon fresh basil, sliced into thin strips

Dash ground black pepper

1 tablespoon feta cheese, grated

Preheat oven to 450 degrees. In skillet, over medium heat 2 teaspoons olive oil and add garlic, onion and zucchini. Cook for approximately 5 minutes. Remove from heat and add tomatoes, basil and pepper. In oven-proof dish, spread 1 tablespoon of olive oil and place halibut on top. Cover fish with mixture and sprinkle with feta cheese. Bake for 12 to 15 minutes or until fish is easily flaked with a fork.

Tenderloin and mushrooms

1 tenderloin steak, cut into strips

1 tablespoon bbq sauce, no sugar added

1 serving organic long whole grain rice

Organic chicken or vegetable broth (for cooking rice)

1 portabella mushroom

1 clove garlic, minced

½ tablespoon butter

Cook rice according to instructions on bag or box. Cut steak into strips. Marinade in bbq sauce. Slice portabella mushrooms. In skillet over medium heat, melt butter. Add garlic and mushrooms. In separate skillet over medium heat add ½ tablespoon of olive oil and cook steak until done to your liking.

Balsamic Chicken Pasta

1 chicken breast, organic or free range (no skin), sliced

1 teaspoon olive oil

1 tablespoon balsamic vinegar

1 clove garlic, minced

⅛ teaspoon basil

⅛ teaspoon oregano

⅛ teaspoon thyme

⅛ teaspoon rosemary

2 or 3 onion slices

1 tomato, diced

Pepper to taste

1 tablespoon serving organic pasta

1 Parmesan cheese

Over medium heat add olive oil, garlic and onion to skillet or wok and add the chicken add the remaining ingredients and cook until chicken is cooked thoroughly. Approximately 12 to 15 minutes. Cook pasta according to directions. Once cooked, mix with chicken dish and sprinkle with Parmesan cheese.

Prawn Stir Fry

8 to 10 tiger prawns

¼ red pepper

¼ yellow pepper

One head baby bok choy

1 cup sprouts

2 stalks celery, sliced

3-4 rings onion, red or white, sliced

2 tablespoons olive oil

1 clove garlic, minced

1 teaspoon Chinese five spice

Over medium heat, heat 1 tablespoon oil and garlic in a wok. Once heated, cook prawns, flipping over half way through. Once cooked remove prawns from the pan. Add additional tablespoon of oil to wok and add onion, celery and peppers. Sprinkle on the Chinese five spice and stir in. Cook for approximately 5 minutes then add baby bok choy, sprouts and cooked prawns and cook for an additional 1 to 2 minutes.

Flatbread

1 serving flatbread, whole grain

½ skinless chicken breast, organic or free range, pulled apart

½ cup cherry tomatoes, chopped

1 clove garlic, minced

¼ cup feta cheese, grated

4 or 5 basil leaves, cut into strips

1 tablespoon olive oil

In oven-safe dish, place chicken and enough chicken or vegetarian broth to halfway cover the breast, and bake at 350 degrees for approximately 22 minutes or until chicken is completely cooked through. In bowl, mix olive oil, garlic, tomatoes, basil and feta cheese together. You can either spread the tomato mixture on the flatbread and top with the chicken or you can mix the chicken into the tomato mixture, whichever you prefer. Bake at 400 degrees for approximately 5 minutes.

Meatloaf

2 eggs, beaten

½ cup organic milk

½ cup whole grain bread crumbs

½ cup onion, finely chopped

2 tablespoons parsley

2 pounds organic lean ground beef

¼ cup of ketchup

2 tablespoons organic brown sugar

1 teaspoon mustard

Mix beef, eggs, milk, breadcrumbs, onion and parsley together and place into baking pan. Bake at 350 degrees for 40 minutes, remove from oven. Mix ketchup, brown sugar and mustard together and cover the top of the meatloaf and bake for an additional 10 minutes.

FOURTH Meal of the Day Options (Liquid Shakes):

The following shakes do not need to have a fat source added, as your nuts and seeds will be your source.

Ultimate Protein of your choice .... 1 serving

Brazil Nuts 4

In a shaker cup, mix Ultimate Protein with water. Eat nuts separately.

Ultimate Protein of your choice .... 1 serving

Cashews 5

Sunflower seeds 12

In a shaker cup mix Ultimate Protein with water. Eat nuts and seeds separately.

Ultimate Protein of your choice .... 1 serving

Almonds 5

Pumpkin seeds 10

Raisins (organic only) 10

In a shaker cup, mix Ultimate Protein with water. Mix nuts and seeds together.

Ultimate Protein of your choice .... 1 serving

Almonds 5

Cashews 4

In a shaker cup, mix Ultimate Protein with water. Eat almonds and cashews separately.

Ultimate Protein of your choice .... 1 serving

Walnuts 5

Almonds 5

In a shaker cup, mix Ultimate Protein with water. Eat walnuts and almonds separately.

Ultimate Protein of your choice .... 1 serving

Pistachios 22

In a shaker cup, mix Ultimate Protein with water. Eat pistachios separately.

Ultimate Protein of your choice .... 1 serving

Sunflower... 12

Pumpkin seeds... 10

In a shaker cup, mix Ultimate Protein with water. Eat sunflower and pumpkin seeds separately.

FIFTH Meal of the Day Options:

Chili

One serving of organic extra-lean ground beef or turkey

½ cup kidney beans

1 or 2 cloves garlic, crushed

¼ onion, diced

1 stalk celery, sliced

1 carrot, sliced

1 Portabello mushroom, cut into cubes

1 glass jar of organic tomato sauce or Arrabbiata sauce (you decide on the consistency that you prefer)

Add chili powder to your taste

In a skillet brown your meat. Once cooked, remove excess fat and add onions and crushed garlic to meat mixture. Cook for approximately 3 minutes. Add tomato sauce, celery, carrot, Portabello mushroom and chili powder. Bring to a boil. Mix well. Cover and simmer for 30 to 45 minutes.

Halibut and Spinach Salad:

1 serving halibut

½ lemon

1 teaspoon olive oil

¼ teaspoon sea salt

1 clove garlic, minced

1 teaspoon oregano

1 serving baby spinach, washed

1 hard boiled egg

1 Portabella mushroom, sliced

1 carrot, grated

2 green onions, sliced

1 avocado, cut into bite-size pieces

Preheat oven to broil. On a baking sheet place tin foil and brush with olive oil. Place halibut on the olive oil. Squeeze the juice from the lemon over fish and sprinkle with sea salt, garlic and oregano. Broil for 12-20 minutes (depending on the thickness of the halibut).

In a large bowl, combine the salad ingredients and toss with a balsamic vinaigrette (ensure there is no sugar in the ingredients) or mix your own using olive oil and balsamic vinegar.

Taco Salad

1 cup romaine lettuce, chopped

1 serving cooked ground turkey

2 tablespoons Havarti cheese with jalapeño, grated

1 tablespoon black olives

¼ red pepper, chopped

¼ yellow pepper, chopped

2 stalks green onion, chopped

½ avocado, chopped

½ cup salsa (or more if you prefer)

Mix all ingredients together.

Salmon Salad:

1 serving romaine lettuce, washed

1 salmon filet

½ tablespoon olive oil

½ tablespoon low-sodium soy sauce

1 clove garlic

½ cup cabbage, shredded

2 or 3 rings of red onion, sliced

1½ tablespoons sliced almonds

Place salmon in baking dish (add a tablespoon of olive oil to dish before placing salmon in it so that the salmon skin does not bake to the dish). In bowl mix ½ tablespoon olive oil, ½ tablespoon low sodium soy sauce and 1 clove of garlic. Mix together and drizzle over salmon. Broil salmon in over for 12-16 minutes (depending on how you like it cooked).

In a large bowl, add lettuce, cabbage, red onion and cooked salmon. Mix together, and sprinkle the sliced almonds on top. Add your choice of salad dressing (no creamy salad dressings allowed!)

Mango/Chicken Salad

2 slices pineapple

2 tablespoons fresh mango, finely chopped

2 rings of red onion, finely chopped

1 tablespoon finely chopped fresh coriander

1 teaspoon fresh lemon juice

2 teaspoon olive oil

1 chicken breast, oven baked and sliced

½ Granny Smith apple, peeled and shredded

1 serving mixed greens, washed

In bowl, place mixed greens and sliced chicken breast, cover with pineapple, mango, red onion, coriander, green apple, lemon juice and olive oil.

I Yam A Steak

1 lean steak, organic if possible

Marinade (see recipe below)

1 cup yam, cut into cubes

1 portabella mushroom, sliced

1½ tablespoon butter, organic

1 clove garlic

Marinade:

1 teaspoon Chinese five spice

2 tablespoons low sodium soy sauce

1 clove garlic, minced

1 tablespoon honey

Cut steak into strips and marinade for 15 minutes to one hour. Over high heat, in a pot bring water to boil and add cubed yam and cook for approximately 8 to 10 minutes or until a knife cleanly cuts through yam. Once cooked, remove from heat, drain and replace in pot. Add ½ tablespoon butter and mash until smooth. Over medium heat in skillet, melt 1 tablespoon butter and add garlic. Add mushrooms and cook until done. Move mushrooms aside or place in separate dish and cook steak over medium heat until done to your liking. Cover the yams with the steak/mushroom mixture.

Avocado/Shrimp Salad

1 serving mixed greens, washed

1 avocado

1 serving hand peeled shrimp

¼ cup broccoli, chopped

1 stalk celery, sliced

6 cherry tomatoes

¼ red pepper, sliced

¼ yellow pepper, sliced

In large bowl, mix mixed greens, celery, cherry tomato's and peppers.

Toss with 1 tablespoon honey mustard dressing. Remove skin and pit from avocado. Cut avocado in half and place equal amounts of shrimp in each avocado. Place this on top of your salad.

Honey Mustard Dressing

¼ cup mayonnaise

1 tablespoon stone ground mustard

1 tablespoon honey

½ tablespoon lemon juice

Chapter Twenty Three:

////////////////// **The Ultimate Male Supplement Protocol**

We are finally at the section I get most excited about – supplementation! As a nutritional researcher, I have formulated numerous nutritional formulas over the years for different companies. I've even been honored for some of these formulations with the Alive Gold Medal of Excellence Award. Having said this, with so many different nutritional formulas and ingredients on the market, I understand how difficult it can be for the untrained person to navigate the nutritional arena. Actually it can be down right confusing at times!

In Chapter Eighteen, I listed a series of nutritional ingredients under varying categories (**Testosterone-Supporting Nutrients**; **Prostate-Protecting Nutrients**; **Libido-Enhancing Nutrients**) in order to give you a perspective on what ingredients have been shown to be highly effective when it comes to aiding in these underlying areas. What I negated to list was recommended dosages, due to the fact that there are numerous variables (i.e. size, weight, lifestyle, stress, etc.) that come into play when it comes to recommended dosages of these nutrients.

Through my many years in the health industry, I also understand that when it comes to actually experiencing results with various nutrients and the formulas they comprise, quality of the ingredients is paramount followed by compliance of taking the ingredients (and formulations) regularly and as per instructions. It is always best if you can find formulations that contain ingredients that have great synergy – in other words, ones that work well and provide greater results by taking them together.

Realizing this fact and having created numerous formulas over the years, I have tried to simplify supplementation by creating cutting-edge formulas that use synergistic ingredients to garnish the greatest results in the least amount of time. These formulas contain many if not all of the recommended ingredients for the varying categories listed in Chapter Eighteen and elsewhere throughout this book. Product information pertaining to each of these formulas can be found at the back of this book.

To make it as easy as possible to follow the supplement portion of **The Ultimate Male Solution**, I have broken your recommended supplement protocol into three parts using my recommended formulations 1) because they have an incredible track record, 2) because they include many of the recommended nutrients and are therefore less expensive than purchasing each ingredient separately and 3) because they are highly effective. The three sections of **The Ultimate Male Solution** supplement protocol are as follows:

Beginner Male: this is for the Weekend Warrior or the beginner who is getting his feet wet and is only interested in dabbling in avoiding or reversing the Beer Belly Blues. Average age – **20-30**

Intermediate Male: this is for the more serious man who wants to take a sober stab at avoiding or reversing the Beer Belly Blues. Average age – **30-45**

Ultimate Male: this is for the no holds barred man who will accept nothing but success at avoiding or reversing the Beer Belly Blues. Average age – **45+**

Your Ultimate Male Supplement Protocol

Beginner Male [Average Age – 20-30]

Formula [or nutrient].. QTY

Ultimate Multi..2 daily with food

Ultimate Male Energy............... 2 twice/daily with or without food

Ultimate Maca.......................... 2 twice/daily with or without food

Protein Isolate ....1 serving 1-2X/daily

Vitamin D3*................................2,000-4,000 IU/daily with food

Fish Oil (molecularly distilled)...............................2,000 mg daily (at least 700 mg EPA, 500 mg DHA)

Intermediate Male [Average Age – 30-45]

Formula [or nutrient]... QTY

Ultimate Multi...2 twice/daily with food

Ultimate Male Energy............... 2 twice/daily with or without food

Ultimate Prostate............................ 1-3 daily with or without food

Ultimate Maca......................... 3 twice/daily with or without food

Ultimate Anti-Stress .... 2 nightly before bed

Ultimate Sleep...1-3 nightly before bed

Protein Isolate ....2 serving daily

Vitamin D3*..4,000 IU/daily with food

Fish Oil (molecularly distilled)...............................2,000 mg daily
(at least 700 mg EPA, 500 mg DHA)

Ultimate Male [Average Age – 45+]

Formula [or nutrient].. QTY

Ultimate Multi...................................... 2-3 twice/daily with food

Ultimate Male Energy............2-3 twice/daily with or without food

Ultimate Prostate............................... 3 daily with or without food

Ultimate Libido .... 3 daily with or without food

Ultimate Maca......................... 4 twice/daily with or without food

Ultimate Anti-Stress .... 2 nightly before bed

Ultimate Sleep...2-3 nightly before bed

Protein Isolate ....2 serving daily

Vitamin D3*..............4,000-7,000 IU (Minimum)/daily with food

Fish Oil (molecularly distilled)...............................2,000 mg daily
(at least 700 mg EPA, 500 mg DHA)

*It is important to closely monitor your vitamin D levels (referred to as 25-Hydroxy Vitamin D), and aim for a blood level of approximately **50 ng/mL**.

Chapter Twenty Four:
Supercharging Biocize

Now that you have become acquainted with the revolutionary form of exercise called Biocize, it's time to put your new exercise protocol into practice. But before you try exercising the Biocize way, it is imperative that you are healthy enough to actually perform high-impact activity by first getting clearance from your medical professional.

Once you have been cleared and are ready to go, make sure you listen carefully to your body – especially during the first few weeks of Biocize – as you don't want to push yourself past the point of being able to recuperate properly. The whole idea behind Biocize is to create the optimal hormonal response in the least amount of time, in order to see fast and consistent results – not to overtrain. This is also why you should make sure to give yourself plenty of rest after Biocize is done, and make sure to take a break from Biocize at least a couple of days each week, as rest is when the body recovers from the exercise and becomes stronger, harder and faster.

When you embark on these types of exercises make sure you give it 100-percent effort during the all-out phases. If you don't, you are only fooling yourself. All-out effort means you will be pushing yourself to the point where it will be extremely difficult, if not next to impossible, to continue past the 20 seconds of all-out effort. In other words you should be praying for that 10-second reprieve, and dreading moving into that 20-second all-out portion again! The beautiful reality to Biocize is it only lasts for the four minutes and you can do anything for four minutes can't you?

Don't Overtrain

If you feel yourself getting weaker or the exercises becoming harder instead of easier for you over time, you could be overtraining. Some of the signs of overtraining include:

- You find it continually difficult to get motivated (you dread working out)

- You stop losing body fat and, in some cases, even gain a little more

- You have trouble sleeping

- You feel anxious or irritable a lot of the time

- Your joints feel inflamed and achy

- You get sick more often

- You feel bad after your workouts

- Your moods have become depressed

If you experience two or three of the above signs, then it is time to lay off the exercise for a while until you start to feel better. Overtraining is one of the easiest ways to obliterate your testosterone levels, so once again listen to your body. In Chapter Seventeen I spoke about the importance of protein and particularly the BCAAs. It turns out that one of the best ways to reduce the possibility of overtraining and ensure recovery from exercise is to maintain high levels of these amino acids both before and after exercising, so pay close attention to what to do both before and after Biocize in order to maximize your results.

Clearing Up the Confusion

Over the years I have been asked too many times to mention about what to consume both before and after exercise. This seems to be one of the most confusing topics to both novice and experienced exercisers. So allow me to clear up any of the confusion so that you are able to concentrate your efforts on doing what needs to get done!

What to Consume Before Biocize

Exercising is stressful on the body, which is why the body responds by elevating certain stress hormones. When the body is stressed, it isn't interested in digesting food. Instead, most of the blood supply is escorted to the extremities, not the stomach. This is why it isn't wise to consume a lot of solid food before exercise; it will just sit there fermenting in your gut. Instead, you should train yourself to either exercise on an empty stomach* (if your exercise first thing in the A.M.), or only consume around 100 calories about 30-45 minutes before the activity. Contrary to popular belief, carbohydrates are not the best things to eat just before training;

they'll raise your insulin levels, causing you to use glucose (sugar) as your primary fuel.

Instead, Biocize exercise dictates that you consume protein. Protein isolates (like whey or sprouted rice) empty from the stomach quickly, but they also cause a rise in the hormone glucagon (the primary hormone for maintaining glucose levels during exercise), which allows for fat-burning activity instead of storage. So if you must eat something before exercise, make it a protein shake with water, and keep it around 100 calories (this would be about one heaping scoop of the Ultimate Protein with one-quarter cup of berries).

If you exercise on an empty stomach, try supplementing with approximately 7 grams of BCAAs about a half-hour prior to starting to Biocize.

What to Consume After Biocize

After any athletic activity, especially Biocize, the body requires refueling of its glycogen (stored sugar in liver and muscles) reserves. In order to ensure this happens, the body contains an enzyme called *glycogen synthetase* that is responsible for storing sugar for future needs. Within 45 minutes-1.5 hours after exercise this enzyme is extra hungry. This is the only time that you can consume larger-than-normal (and higher glycemic) amounts of carbohydrates without worrying that they'll convert to fat.

Many of us usually make the mistake of consuming only carbohydrates at this time (juice, etc.). This is wrong! Drinking carbohydrate beverages without sufficient protein after Biocize will cause a drastic increase in insulin levels, bringing the increase in growth hormone and testosterone levels to a halt. Studies confirm that protein mixed with carbohydrates after training allows for faster muscle recovery and greater growth hormone and testosterone increases. Always mix protein with carbohydrates – such as fresh or frozen berries – as close to completing your workout as possible to ensure rapid replacement of bodily sugars and protein for recovery. The post-Biocize protein should be primarily in the form of high alpha-lactalbumin whey protein isolate for maximum timing and absorption value as well as it's extremely high levels of BCAAs. Once again, the carbohydrates should come from mixed whole fruits, primarily from the berry family due to their superior antioxidant-carrying capacity.

The Importance of Water

During exercise, it's imperative to increase your water intake due to its vital role in cardiovascular function and temperature regulation. As you exercise, your body loses a great deal of water through sweating and evaporation, and your muscles create a lot of extra heat. The heat is transported through tiny blood vessels called capillaries near the surface of your skin. The release of perspiration (and its evaporation) from your sweat glands creates a cooling effect on the skin as well as the blood in the capillaries beneath it. Sweating is therefore an essential part of your body's cooling system.

If your body does not have enough water to make this system run smoothly, your blood-carrying capacity also diminishes. Don't forget, it is the blood's role to carry nutrients such as oxygen, glucose, fatty acids and proteins to the muscles to create energy. The blood must also remove the toxic elements of metabolism, such as carbon dioxide. Since your circulatory system is almost 70 percent water, the extra demand on it can be quite severe.

Intensive exercise can cause a person to lose 5-8 pounds of fluid through perspiration, evaporation and exhalation. Studies show that for every pound of fluid lost, there is a significant drop in the efficiency with which the body produces energy. In one study, a 4 percent loss of body weight from exercise-induced dehydration resulted in 31 percent shorter muscle-endurance time. It's amazing to think that something as simple as water can be the determining factor in winning or losing a competition. Many studies also point out the importance of proper hydration in managing the oxidative stress load of exercise due to the overproduction of those nasty little free radicals. Still other research indicates proper hydration in protecting and modulating our immune response to exercise.

Try to consume clean filtered water throughout the day

Losing excess fat can cause a release of toxins into your body, since many toxins become lodged in the fatty tissue. Water is essential in the detoxification process, and since you will be dropping fat like mad, you will need all you can drink.

As pointed out in one of my earlier books, *Bio-Age: 10 Steps to a Younger You*, the late Dr. Batmanghelidj presented an interesting theory that somewhere through our evolution the signals for thirst and hunger may have become one and the same. Dr. Batmanghelidj believed that often when we think we are hungry we are, in fact, just thirsty. So in order to cut down on the urge to overeat, it is recommended that you drink a glass of water before eating. This way you will be guaranteed not to overeat to satisfy an urge for water intake. Carry your water with you in a closed container everywhere you go (I even bring my water to bed) and drink it through a straw to avoid ingesting excess air.

If you have never worked out in this manner before, or have never worked out period, I highly advise that you get yourself a qualified personal trainer to show you the ropes – and don't forget to first clear it with your health professional. Welcome to the new realm of Biocize exercise; welcome to the newer, younger YOU.

Chapter Twenty Five:

Hormone Testing for the Ultimate Male

Whether we're talking about sex drive or overall prostate health, nothing is more important for men than overall testosterone levels. Whether due to internal body processes or external environmental factors, the loss of testosterone is troubling for men concerned about their health. As you are now well aware, low testosterone is a hallmark of the Beer Belly Blues.

As a brief recap: lower testosterone levels have been scientifically linked to a number of moderate-to-severe issues, including:

- Muscle loss
- Weight gain (increase in body fat)
- Bone density loss (osteoporosis)
- Hair loss
- Insomnia and/or disruptions in normal sleep patterns
- Loss of interest in sex
- Depression
- Erectile dysfunction (difficulty achieving and/or maintaining an erection)
- Difficulty with concentration/memory
- Loss of energy
- Increased risk for cardiovascular disease

Without question, the loss of testosterone can have very serious consequences for a man's physical, mental and sexual health. The good news is you are now well-armed in various tactics of combating testosterone loss through effective lifestyle, diet, exercise and supplementation protocols. Each of the strategies discussed in this book – especially when combined – can help enhance existing testosterone levels, reduce the level of natural age-related loss, and even help alleviate symptoms.

The first step in the process is to find out if you are presently experiencing less than adequate levels of testosterone. In order to know for sure (besides the many obvious signs listed throughout this book), you'll need to have your testosterone level checked.

Who should consider having testosterone levels tested?

Any man over age 35, or any man experiencing one or more of the symptoms listed above should have their testosterone tested on a regular basis.

Testing Options – Blood vs. Salivary

In a laboratory setting, blood tests are most common and usually involve a small sample taken from the arm in the early morning when testosterone levels are highest. However, do-it-yourself at home tests are also available and measure levels in the saliva (salivary tests). For anyone experiencing symptoms of the Beer Belly Blues, the blood test is definitely recommended. But for anyone just looking to monitor testosterone levels as they age, the saliva tests can help identify emerging problems. Users simply have to collect saliva at specified times during the day and then mail the sample to the lab or the company providing the test. Results usually take two to three weeks.

What If Testosterone Replacement Is Required?

In some cases of low testosterone, a qualified health professional may recommend a regimen of testosterone therapy using prescription-only products. In this case it is always best to discuss bio-identical testosterone replacement with your physician.

Bio-identical testosterone is best taken as a topically applied cream purchased from a compounding pharmacy. These compounded testosterone creams are able to supply the same testosterone produced in your body at precise amounts that are easily absorbed into the bloodstream. This is also the best way to approximate the way testosterone is naturally produced – or at least should be – by the body each day. Compounded testosterone creams are much less expensive than brand-name testosterone creams or gels. (NOTE: in some instances – as determined by your physician – testosterone injections are the next best choice versus topically applied creams.)

It is always wise to avoid oral ingestion of testosterone in the form of pills, as oral testosterone is quickly degraded by liver enzymes, which more often than not leads to unhealthy variations in blood levels of testosterone and possible liver problems. This in no way reflects upon the use of the natural research-proven ingredients (nutrients) I mentioned in this book, as those help combat low testosterone in natural ways.

Recommended Male Panel Tests

Blood and salivary tests are the two basic options for testosterone testing, but there are several other specific male panel tests to consider, including:

- Free Testosterone (Total Testosterone)
- Estradiol
- Pregnenolone
- DHEA Sulfate
- Lipid Profile
- TSH (Thyroid Stimulating Hormone)
- PSA (Total and Free)
- CRP (C-Reactive Protein)
- 25-Hydroxy Vitamin D

Testing Overview

The following is a brief overview of each test.

Free Testosterone (Total Testosterone)

As I mentioned in Chapter Eleven: Not All Testosterone is Created Equal, it is extremely important to understand that testosterone exists in two primary forms in the body: free and bound. Free testosterone refers to the amount of the sex hormone actually available to the body for use — that is, it is not bound. Testosterone can be bound by either Albumin (a serum protein) or Sex Hormone Binding Globulin (SHBG). Albumin is considered a rather weak binding agent that the body can easily break, and therefore it uses most testosterone that is bound to it. SHBG, on the other hand, forms a strong bond that is very difficult for the body to break so any testosterone bound to it is not considered to be free or usable by the body.

Unfortunately, many testosterone tests measure the total testosterone present in the blood, which includes both free and bound versions. This does not present a clear picture of how much testosterone is actually available to the body and is therefore not considered to be a comprehensive measure of existing levels. An equilibrium dialysis test is considered superior to a total test because it measures free testosterone plus a portion of the albumin-bound testosterone while excluding any hormones bound to SHBG. This is a much clearer indication of the amount of testosterone available to the body for use, but the costs of this test are greater. However, to get the clearest picture possible of "usable" testosterone, the added costs are well worth it.

It is also wise to know what your SHBG levels are, as I pointed out in that same chapter, high SHBG levels correlate to lower testosterone. However, extremely low levels are just as bad and can contribute greatly to diseases associated with age.

So what results should you hope for with a testosterone and a SHBG test? That answer actually depends on a lot of factors. But remember, blood-test laboratory reference ranges are age adjusted, reflecting the anticipated reduction in testosterone that almost all men experience.

This is why I have listed what are referred to as "optimal ranges", which reflect what an average man would produce in his twenties or early thirties. As it pertains to testosterone, optimum levels should be near the higher end of that range.

The following are considered normal/healthy ranges for most men:

- **Total Testosterone:** between **350-1200 ng/dL** (optimal levels lean towards the upper range as long as free testosterone is above **20 pg/mL**)
- **Free Testosterone:** 20-25 pg/mL or **higher**
- **Sex Hormone Binding Globulin (SHBG):** between **30-40 nmol/L**

Estradiol

As you read in Chapter 12: Estradiol – What You Need to Know, estradiol is a form of estrogen (actually it is the primary estrogen from which all other estrogens are made) and is considered to be primarily a female hormone, though it is found in both men and women. For men, levels increase when testosterone is converted into estrogen via the aromatase enzyme. Elevated levels of estradiol have been associated with increased risk for prostate cancer, while extremely low levels can increase the risk of bone fractures and lower bone density. Because it is so important to male health for estradiol levels not to be too high or low, testing is increasingly vital as men experiencing the Beer Belly Blues age due to the increased fluctuations of this hormone.

Optimal levels of estradiol should be between: **20-30 pg/mL**

Note: men who experience high levels of estradiol may need to use aromatase-inhibiting nutrients (i.e. chrysin) or drugs (such as Arimidex®: 0.5mg/twice per week) to bring their levels back into a healthier range.

Pregnenolone

Although it may be difficult to locate a facility that tests pregnenolone levels, this hormone actually plays a huge role in the aging process. Pregnenolone is actually a building block vital to the production of several other important hormones, including: testosterone, DHEA, estrogen and progesterone. But just as with overall testosterone levels, the body begins producing less and less pregnenolone beginning in the early to mid-30s. For men facing andropause, pregnenolone is an important ally because it is likely to be converted into testosterone if levels are low. Pregnenolone is also useful in fighting other problems associated with aging, such as fatigue and poor memory. Studies even show it can stimulate brain-cell growth.

Optimal levels of pregnenolone should be between: **100-170 ng/dL**

DHEA-S (sulfate)

Perhaps ironically, DHEA levels are typically only tested when an excess of testosterone is suspected because it can indicate the presence of tumors in the adrenal gland. However, because testosterone is also produced in the adrenal glands, testing for DHEA is also important for anyone facing the Beer Belly Blues or any of its symptoms. Low levels of DHEA can indicate a problem in adrenal-gland function (including high cortisol) and a potential source of low testosterone levels.

Optimal levels of DHEA-S should be between: **350-490 μg/dL**

TSH (Thyroid Stimulating Hormone)

The TSH test basically assesses thyroid gland function, which affects growth, development, and body metabolism. Hypothyroidism (low thyroid function is signified by the production of too much TSH, and can produce symptoms that resemble many andropause issues, including loss of energy, muscle weakness, depression, hair loss and weight gain. Hypothyroidism has also been linked with increased risk for cardiovascular disease.

Even though TSH readings are considered normal at levels up to **5.5 mU/L**, research indicates that the optimal range of **TSH is below 2.0 mU/L.**

Lipid Profile

As the name suggests, a lipid profile does not really look at testosterone levels. Rather, it looks at total cholesterol, HDL, LDL and triglycerides. Having said this, numerous studies do indicate that HDL levels are directly correlated to those of testosterone (i.e. higher HDL = higher testosterone levels).

The purpose of a lipid profile is ultimately to determine the risk for coronary artery disease. Low testosterone levels have been linked with increased risk of coronary artery disease, so a lipid profile is merely a precautionary test usually performed in conjunction with a testosterone test and will likely be recommended by your physician. A lipid profile is definitely recommended for anyone who:

- Smokes cigarettes/tobacco products
- Is over the age of 45 for men, 55 for women
- Has hypertension (blood pressure above 140/90)
- Has a family history of coronary heart disease

The total cholesterol/HDL ratio is much more important as an overall cholesterol measurement – when it comes to cardiovascular risk – than TC (total cholesterol) is. In order to calculate the total cholesterol/HDL ratio, the total cholesterol value is divided by the value of the HDL cholesterol. (High ratios indicate higher risks of heart attacks, low ratios indicate lower risk).

An acceptable ratio of TC/HDL is **4.5 or below** (however **below 4.0** is much more desirable).

PSA (Total and Free)

Prostate Specific Antigen (PSA) is a protein produced naturally in the prostate gland. Elevated levels may be an indication of problems in the prostate, particularly prostate cancer. Many physicians believe that a PSA test is vital, though it is important to note that the PSA has one of the highest false-positive rates of any medical test – as high as 85 percent. In fact, one well-controlled study that appeared in the *New England Journal of Medicine* (1991) showed that 78 percent of men who scored high on the PSA (between 4-10), showed no trace of cancer when subjected to a biopsy.

The total PSA test should be used in conjunction with a digital rectal exam (DRE) and is often performed on men already suffering with prostate cancer to help verify the effectiveness of treatment. However, a total PSA can also be used on patients with prostate cancer symptoms, such as difficult, painful and/or infrequent urination, as well as back pain and pelvic pain. Most doctors will recommend a biopsy when elevated levels of PSA are indicated, though you should always ask for a second or third opinion before going this route. The total PSA is currently believed to be the best way to assess prostate health without a biopsy, and the American Cancer Association recommends an annual total PSA test for men starting at age 50.

A healthy PSA reading is **below 4.0 ng/mL**, with free-PSA **above 25 percent** (free-PSA is lower in people with prostate cancer).

CRP (C-Reactive Protein)

The CRP test is used to help assess overall heart health, which is a major concern for men with low testosterone levels, as the test can help determine an increased risk for coronary heart disease. Aside from this it is also a very effective measure of overall inflammation in the body (inflammation is one of the key causes of coronary heart disease).

Crohn's disease, or inflammatory bowel disease, is another problem men face as they get older. Elevated CRP levels indicate the presence of infection or inflammation, so testing for this protein can help identify potential problems with intestinal disorders, as well.

Normally, levels of CRP hover **around 4.9mg/L**, but the optimal level of CRP in your blood would be **under 2mg/L**. The presence of an infection or inflammation can send the reading above 100mg/L. making it easy to identify a potential problem.

25-Hydroxy Vitamin D Test

At the beginning of Part III you learned how important the sunshine vitamin is when it comes to supporting optimal testosterone levels, so it only makes sense to find out what your vitamin D status is in order to get it to the level it needs to be. The 25-hydroxy vitamin D test is the most accurate way that you can measure how much vitamin D is in your body.

Aim for a blood level of approximately **50 ng/mL**.

Various Testosterone Treatments

Below I have listed the various testosterone treatments that are available by prescription along with the **approximate recommended dosages** for each treatment. **Please check with a qualified health professional before exploring any of these options as each individual treatment is unique and should be CLOSELY MONITORED.**

- **Compounded Creams:** 100mg/day

- **Injections [cypionate and enanthate]:** 100-400mg/every 2 weeks

- **Patches [Androderm® – account for 12 percent of market]:** 44 percent of users have skin irritations. Applied to lower abdomen

- **Gels [AndroGel® & Testim® – account for 60 percent of market]:** 5-10g applied once/day to upper arm, shoulders or chest. 15-20 percent of men do not absorb them well or at all.

- **Pellets [Testopel® – extended-release]:** 6-8 pellets (size of a grain of rice) injected under the skin (buttocks). Lasts 3-6 months.

- **Buccal Treatment [Striant®]:** adhesive pellet applied to the upper gum twice/day.

All of the tests mentioned above – with the exception of the pregnenolone test – are vital to men and can help identify potential health problems relating to testosterone loss in time to treat them. While not all tests look specifically at testosterone, or even hormone levels, all of the Male Panel Tests mentioned here will help promote male health by identifying potential problems associated with aging, including andropause. Once again, I have listed the optimal ranges of each test based on the latest studies, however only a qualified health professional can assess your personal levels effectively.

The most important tests of all are, of course, those that test for free and total testosterone due to the fact that testosterone is the elixir of life and health for men, and testing for it should be an integral part of health maintenance and care.

Appendix I

////////////////////////// **The Ultimate Male Way to Supplement**

In Parts, II and III of **The Ultimate Male Solution**, I described various nutrients that offer special benefits where overall health – especially male health – is concerned. Many of these nutrients can be found in synergistic combinations within special formulas mentioned below.

What Constitutes a Great Product?

From my many years in the health industry, I have come to realize that a nutrient formula is only as good as the quality of its starting ingredients and the manufacturing practices used to create it. Therefore it is imperative to cover all the bases when creating a high-quality nutrient formula. Following is the criteria I have used as a product formulator over the years:

- There must be a real need for the specific product

- All ingredients within the formula must be of the highest quality

- All ingredients within the formula need to be researched based and in the ratios and/or extracts found in the studies that support their efficacy

- All ingredients within the formula need to work in synergy

- Each new production batch must be third-party verified for quality assurance

I guarantee that all products in the Ultimate line meet the above criteria and are among the best – if not the best – products in the industry.

Note: Most of the recommended supplements in this section can be found throughout Canada at local health food retailers. If you reside outside of Canada, you can find these formulas online at **www.AwakenYourBody. com**. We do not sell online to Canadians because we are committed to supporting the health food stores in which these products are carried.

All Ultimate products are distributed (exclusively through health food stores) in Canada by:

Preferred Nutrition, Inc.

Order Desk: 1-888-826-9625

Fax: 1-888-773-7069

www.pno.ca

Outside Canada:

Online only: **www.AwakenYourBody.com**

Following is a brief description of each recommended formula. Under each formula you will find a list of ingredients that are mentioned in Chapter Eighteen. Not all of the ingredients found in the formula are listed here. For more information on each formula, including *all* ingredients and dosages, please visit **www.AwakenYourBody.com** and click on the products icon.

Ultimate High-Alpha Whey Protein™

The Ultimate High-Alpha Whey Protein™ is a one-of-a-kind, high-performance, functional protein that contains the highest levels of the bioactive peptide Alpha-lactalbumin – nature's most perfect form of protein. The exceptionally high levels of bioactive proteins, peptides and amino acids are obtained through an exclusive low-heat, cross-flow micro-filtration method that filters out all impurities and guarantees a completely bioavailable protein coming from 100 percent whey isolate (no inexpensive, less bioavailable concentrate). The result is a protein that can actually impact the body's biological systems and help lower stress hormones (cortisol), balance moods, reduce cravings, aid in deep restorative sleep (i.e. supporting optimal HGH production) and boost energy levels during the day. **Ultimate High-Alpha Whey Protein™** is guaranteed to contain a minimum of 33 percent Alpha-lactalbumin.

The unique levels of bioactive proteins, peptides and amino acids in Ultimate **High-Alpha Whey Protein™** play a number of significant health-enhancing roles in the body, some of which include (but are not limited to):

- building, repairing and replacing body cells for faster recuperation
- building and repairing muscle, skin and bones
- reducing appearance of wrinkles
- promoting healthy hair and nails
- improving metabolism (i.e. fat loss)
- balancing immunity for greater defense against disease
- effectively reducing stress
- effectively lowering cortisol
- enhancing feel-good brain chemicals (serotonin)
- aiding in efficient sleep

Ultimate Multi Maximum-Performance™

The **Ultimate Multi Maximum-Performance™** is the most complete multi vitamin/mineral formula available today. The formula contains optimal daily levels of all essential nutrients in their most bioavailable forms. There truly is no other multi vitamin/mineral formula that can compare in quality or value.

Ultimate Male Energy™

Ultimate Male Energy™ contains a synergistic blend of the following 100-percent natural ingredients:

- Chrysin
- Stinging Nettle Root
- Indole-3-Carbinol
- Bioperine® (black pepper extract)

The formula helps restore healthy, youthful hormone balance by positively affecting both estrogen and testosterone production.

Ultimate Prostate™

Ultimate Prostate™ contains a synergistic blend of the following 100-percent natural ingredients:

- Beta sitosterol (non-genetically modified)

- Stinging Nettle Root
- Lycopene
- Indole-3-Carbinol
- Zinc (Aminomin™)
- Bioperine® (black pepper extract)

The formula helps restore healthy prostate function and reduce urinary frequency (BPH) by blocking harmful DHT levels as well as reducing harmful estrogens (and their metabolites).

Ultimate Libido™

Ultimate Libido™ contains a synergistic blend of the following 100-percent natural ingredients:

- Tongkat Ali (100:1 extract from Malaysia)
- Epimedium
- Zinc (Aminomin™)
- Bioperine® (black pepper extract)

The formula helps enhance all facets of libido by naturally working to elevate levels of free testosterone.

Ultimate Maca Energy™

Ultimate Maca Energy™ contains 100 percent certified organic Peruvian Maca that has had its fiber and starch removed through a unique gelatinization process to maximize absorption and bioavailability.

Ultimate Anti-Stress™

Ultimate Anti-Stress™ contains a synergistic blend of the following 100-percent natural ingredients:

- Ashwagandha Extract
- Valerian Extract
- Citrus Bioflavonoids
- Lyophilized Adrenal Tissue
- Quercetin

- Rhodiola Extract

- Bioperine® (black pepper extract)

The formula helps restore healthy adrenal function by working to lower excess cortisol levels. Cortisol competes with testosterone, so **Ultimate Anti-Stress™** is a testosterone-supportive formula.

Ultimate Sleep™

Ultimate Sleep™ contains a synergistic blend of the following 100-percent natural ingredients:

- 5-HTP (from Griffonia simplicifolia)

- Melatonin

- Jujube (Zizyphus jujuba) fruit

- L-Theanine

- L-Lysine

- Niacinamide

- Bioperine® (black pepper extract)

This is one of the most advanced sleep-supporting formulas available today. It combines serotonin-enhancing ingredients along with anti-anxiety/calming nutrients with low-dose melatonin for deep-sleep support.

Natural Cholesterol-Lowering Alternatives

In Chapter Fourteen, **The Truth about Statins**, I recommended a couple of ingredients that are incredible natural alternatives to the harsh, side-effect laden medications that are prescribed like candy these days for lowering cholesterol. Both of these incredible research-proven formulas can be found through **www.pno.ca**.

ImmunoCare™

ImmunoCare™ contains a synergistic blend of the following 100-percent natural ingredients:

- Plant sterols (non-genetically modified)

- Cellasate™

- Enzogenol™
- Essential fatty Acids

Consumption of plant sterols 15 minutes prior to a meal helps block the intestinal absorption of cholesterol. Recent studies have shown that both phytosterols and Enzogenol can assist in reducing LDL, and in increasing HDL levels. In fact, the United States FDA issued a rare ruling allowing the health claim that foods containing plant sterols may reduce cholesterol levels. This is only the 12th time the FDA has allowed such a claim.

Sytrinol®

Sytrinol® contains a synergistic blend of the following 100-percent natural ingredients:

- Mandarin Orange Extract (containing 36 percent Polymethoxylated Flavones)
- Palm Extract (containing 15 percent Tocotrienols)

Clinical trials have shown that Sytrinol acts synergistically to improve total cholesterol by 30 percent, lower LDL cholesterol by 27 percent, and reduce triglycerides by 34 percent (compared to a placebo). Sytrinol has also been shown to increase HDL levels.

References

Part I

Chapter 1:
The Male Transition

Falloon, W. Startling Low Testosterone Blood Levels in Male Life Extension Members. Life Extension Magazine June 2010

Chapter 2:
Your Life on Testosterone

Moncada, Ignacio. Testosterone and Men's Quality of Life. The Aging Male, December 2006; 9(4): 189–193

Shores, M., et al. Low serum testosterone and mortality in male veterans. Arch Intern med. 2006 Aug 14-28;166(15):1660-5.

Chapter 3:
Your Energy on Testosterone

Brunner C, Wuillemin WA. Iron deficiency and iron deficiency anemia - symptoms and therapy. Ther Umsch. 2010 May;67(5):219-23.

Gettler, Lee. Fatherhood, Childcare, and Testosterone: Study Authors Discuss the Details. Scientific American. October 5 2011.

"Male Menopause: Myth or Reality?." Mayo Foundation for Medical Education and Research. (2011): n. page. Web. 20 Jan. 2012. <http://www.mayoclinic.com/health/male-menopause/MC00058>.

Morales A. Testosterone replacement: when is there a role? Int J Impot Res. 2000 Oct;12 Suppl 4:S112-8.

Penev PD. Association between sleep and morning testosterone levels in older men. Sleep, 2007 Apr;30(4):427-32.

ThirdAge.com. Low Testosterone Levels Restrict Deep Sleep. May 21, 2010

Chapter 4:
Your Belly on Testosterone

Allan CA, et al. Body composition, metabolic syndrome and testosterone in ageing men. Int J Impot Res. 2007 Sep;19(5):448-57.

Arver, S, and M Lehtithet. "Current Guidelines for the Diagnosis of Testosterone Deficiency." Front Horm Res. 37. (2009): 5-20. Web. 20 Jan. 2012.

De Pergola G. The adipose tissue metabolism: role of testosterone and dehydroepiandrosterone. Int J Obes Relat Metab Disord. 2000 Jun;24 Suppl 2S59-S63.

Folsom A, Stevens J. "Body Mass Index, Waist/Hip Ratio, and Coronary Heart Disease Incidence in African Americans and Whites." American Journal of Epidimiology. 148.12 (1998): 1187-95. Print.

Grossman, M, EJ Gianetti, et al. "Testosterone and Type 2 Diabetes." Current Opinion Endocrinology Diabetes Obesity. 17.3 (2010): 247-56. Print.

Phillips, GB. "Relationship Between Serum Sex Hormones and the Glucose-insulin-lipid Defect in Men with Obesity." Department of Medicine Columbia University. 42.1 (1993): 116-20. Web. 20 Jan. 2012.

Rebuffe-Scrive M, Marin P, Bjorntorp P. Effect of testosterone on abdominal adipose tissue in men. Int J Obes. 1991 Nov;15(11):791-5.

Stanworth, Roger, and T Hughes Jones. "Testosterone for the Aging Male; Current Evidence and Recommended Practice." PubMed. (2008): n. page. Print.

Svartberg J, et al. Waist Circumference and Testosterone Levels in Community

Swelling Men – the Tromso Study. Eur J Epidemiol. 2004;19(7):657-63.

Chapter 5:
Your Muscles on Testosterone

Delev, DP, , et al. "Physiological and Clinical Characterisitics of Andropause." Folia Med (Plovdiv). 51.1 (2009): 15-22.

Fujita S, Volpi E. Amino acids and muscle loss with aging. J Nutr. 2006 Jan;136(1 Suppl):277S–80S.

Griggs, RC, and W Kingston. "Effect of Testosterone on Muscle Mass and Muscle Protein Synthesis." Journal of Applied Physiology. 66.1 (1989): 498-503. Print.

Layman DK. The role of leucine in weight loss diets and glucose homeostasis. J Nutr. 2003 Jan;133(1):261S-267S.

Yeap, BB. "Testosterone and Ill-Health in Aging Men." Nat Clin Pract Endocrinol Metab. 5.2 (2009): 113-21.

Chapter 6:
Your Brain on Testosterone

Almeida OP, et al. Low free testosterone concentration as a potentially treatable cause of depressive symptoms in older men. Arch Gen Psychiatry. 2008 Mar;65(3):283-9.

Barrett-Connor, E, et al. "Endogenous Sex Hormones and Cognitive Funcrtion in Older Men." J Clin Endocrinol. 84.10 (1999)

Barrett-Connor E, et al. Bioavailable testosterone and depressed mood in older men: the Rancho Bernardo Study. J Clin Endocrinol Metab 1999; 84:573-77.

Hogervorst, Eva, et al. "Serum Total Testosterone is Lower in Men with Alzheimer's ." Neuroendocrinology Letters. 22. (2001): 163-68. Print.

Morley, JE, E Charlton. "Validation of a Screening Questionnaire for Androgen Deficiency in Aging Males." Metabolism. 49.9 (2000): 1239-42. Print.

Young, Laura, Michelle Neiss. "Cognition is Not Modified by Large but Temporary Changes in Sex Hormones in Men." Endocrine Society. (2010)

Chapter 7:
Your Heart on Testosterone

Alberti KG, et al. Harmonizing the metabolic syndrome: a joint interim statement of the International Diabetes Federation Task Force on Epidemiology and Prevention: National Heart, Lung, and Blood Institute; American Heart Association; World Heart Federation; International Atherosclerosis Society; and International Association for the Study of Obesity. Circulation. 2009;120:1640-1645.

Phillips, GB. "Relationship Between Serum Sex Hormones and the Glucose-insulin-lipid Defect in Men with Obesity." Department of Medicine Columbia University. 42.1 (1993): 116-20.

Stanworth, Roger. "Testosterone for the Aging Male; Current Evidence and Recommended Practice." PubMed. (2008)

Traish, AM, F Saad. "The Dark Side of Testosterone Deficiency: III. Cardiovascular Disease." J Androl. 30.5 (2009): 477-94.

Yeap, BB. "Testosterone and Ill-Health in Aging Men." Nat Clin Pract Endocrinol Metab. 5.2 (2009): 113-21.

Chapter 8:
Your Blood Sugar on Testosterone

Arver, S, et al. "Current Guidelines for the Diagnosis of Testosterone Deficiency." Front Horm Res. 37. (2009): 5-20.

"BMI Classification". World Health Organization.

Dhindsa S, et al. Frequent occurrence of hypogonadotropic hypogonadism in type 2 diabetes. J Clin Endocrinol Metab. 2004 Nov;89(11):5462-8.

E.g., the Body Mass Index Table from the National Institutes of Health's NHLBI.

Goepp, Julius. "Low Testosterone Promotes Abdominal Obesity in Aging Men." Life Extension Magazine. Oct 2010: Web.

Grossman, M, EJ Gianetti, et al. "Testosterone and Type 2 Diabetes." Current Opinion Endocrinology Diabetes Obesity. 17.3 (2010): 247-56.

Haffner, SM, , et al. "Insulin Resistance, Body Fat Distribution, and Sex Hormones in Men." Diabetes. 43.2 (1994): 212-9.

Kalyani RR, Dobs AS. Androgen deficiency, diabetes, and the metabolic syndrome in men. Curr Opin Endocrinol Diabetes Obes. 2007 Jun;14(3):226-34.

McGlothin, P, Averill M. Glucose Control: The Sweet Spot in Longevity. The CR Way: Using the Secrets of Calorie Restriction for a Longer, Healthier Life. NY: HarperCollins; 2008:57-78.

Norman, J. "Normal Regulation of Blood Glucose: The Important Roles of Insulin and Glucagon: Diabetes and Hypoglycemia." EndocrinWeb. Web. 27 Jan. 2012.

Ryan, GJ, and LJ Jobe. "Age-Related Androgen Deficiency and Type 2 Diabetes." J Pharm Pract. 24.3 (2011): 316-22.

Singer-Vine, Jeremy. Beyond BMI: Why doctors won't stop using an outdated measure for obesity. State.com, July 20, 2009

Testosterone patch to beat diabetes. Diabetes News – Diabetes.co.uk, Tue, 06 Apr 2010

Chapter 9:
Your Unit on Testosterone

Billups KL, et al. Erectile Dysfunction Is a Marker for Cardiovascular Disease: Results of the Minority Health Institute Expert Advisory Panel. The Journal of Sexual Medicine. Volume 2 Issue 1 Page 40 - January 2005

Gore, J, and J Raifer . " "The Role of Serum Testosterone Testing: Routine Hormone Analysis in an Essential Part of the Initial Screening of Men with Erectile Dysfunction"." Rev Urol. 6.4 (2004): 201-10.

Kim, JW, and D Moon. ""Diagnosis and Treatment of Sexual Dysfunctions in Late-Onset Hypogonadism"." Korean J Urol. 52.11 (2011): 725-35.

Kratzik, CW, , et al. ""The Impact of Age, Body Mass Index and Testosterone on Erectile Dysfunction"." J Urol. 174.1 (2005): 240-7.

Ponholzer, A, et al. ""Prevalence and Risk Factors for Erectile Dysfunction in 2869 Men Using a Validated Questionnaire"."

Eur Urol . 47.1 (2005): 80-5.

Zhang XH, et al. Testosterone restores diabetes-induced erectile dysfunction and sildenafil responsiveness in two distinct animal models of chemical diabetes. J Sex Med. 2006 Mar;3(2):253-266

Chapter 10:
Your Prostate on Testosterone

American Cancer Society website. www. cancer.org

Burnet NG, et al. Normal tissue radiosensitivity – how important is it? Clin Oncol (R Coll Radiol). 1996;8(1):25-34.

Collins MM, et al. "How common is prostatitis? A national survey of physician visits". J Urol. 1998 Apr;159(4):1224-8.

Fang YZ, Yang S, Wu G. Free radicals, antioxidants, and nutrition. Nutrition. 2002 Oct;18(10):872-9.

Gann PH, et al. A prospective evaluation of plasma prostate-specific antigen for detection of prostatic cancer. JAMA. 1995 Jan 25;273(4):289-94.

Hankey, BF; et al. "Cancer surveillance series: interpreting trends in prostate cancer—part I: Evidence of the effects of screening in recent prostate cancer incidence, mortality, and survival rates". J Natl Cancer Inst. (June 16 1999) 91 (12): 1017–24.

Hellerstedt BA, Pienta KJ (2002). The current state of hormonal therapy for prostate cancer. CA—A Cancer Journal for Clinicians, 52: 154–179.

Hsing AW, Chokkalingam AP. "Prostate cancer epidemiology". Frontiers in Bioscience (2006) 11: 1388–413.

Isom-Batz, G, FJ Bianco, et al. "Testosterone as a Predictor of Pathological Stage in Clinically Localized Prostate Cancer." J Urol. 173.6 (2005): 1935-7.

Morgentaler, A, and CO Brunning. "Occult Prostate Cancer in Men withLow Serum Testosterone Levels." JAMA. 276.23 (1996): 1904-6.

"Prostatitis: Benign Prostate Disease: Merck Manual Professional." http://bit.ly/yXLmEp

"ACS :: What Is Prostate Cancer?"

American Cancer Society :: Information and Resources for Cancer: Breast, Colon, Prostate, Lung and Other. http://bit.ly/zQjMdD.

Smith WA, et al. Effect of chemopreventive agents on DNA adduction induced by the potent mammary carcinogen dibenzo[a,l]opyrene in the human breast cells MCF-7. Mutat Res. 2001 Sep 1;480-481:97-108.

van der Cruijsen-Koeter, IW, et al. "Comparison of screen detected and clinically diagnosed prostate cancer in the European randomized study of screening for prostate cancer, section rotterdam". Urol. (July, 2005) 174 (1): 121–5.

Zeegers MP; Jellema, A; Ostrer, H. "Empiric risk of prostate carcinoma for relatives of patients with prostate carcinoma: a meta-analysis". Cancer (2003) 97 (8): 1894–903. .

//

Part II

Chapter 11:
Not All Testosterone is Created Equal

Adams JS. "Bound" to work: the free hormone hypothesis revisited. Cell. 2005 Sep 9;122(5):647-9.

Caldwell JD, Jirikowski GF. Sex hormone binding globulin and aging. Horm Metab Res. 2009 Mar;41(3):173-82.

Clark,AF, et al. Plasma testosterone free index: a better indicator of plasma androgen activity? Fertil Steril. 1975 Oct;26(10):1001-5.

Chuang, AC, et al. "Albuminuria is an Independent Risk Factor of Erectile Dysfunction in Men with Type 2 Diabetes." J Sex Med. (2012): Web. 1 Feb. 2012.

Chubb SA, et al. Lower sex hormone-binding globulin is more strongly associated with metabolic syndrome than lower total testosterone in older men: the Health in Men Study. Eur J Endocrinol. 2008 Jun;158(6):785-92.

Hammond, GL, et al. "Sex Hormone-Binding Globulin: Gene Organization and Structure/Function Analyses." Horm Res. 45.3-5 (1996): 197-201.

Kalme T, et al. Sex hormone-binding globulin and insulin-like growth factor-binding protein-1 as indicators of metabolic syndrome, cardiovascular risk, and mortality in elderly men. J Clin Endocrinol Metab. 2005 Mar;90(3):1550-6.

Ly, LP, et al. "Empirical estimation of free testosterone from testosterone and sex hormone-binding globulin immunoassays." Eur J Endocrinol. 152.3 (2005): 471-8. Print.

Morris, PD, CJ Malkin, et al. "A mathematical comparison of techniques to predict biologically available testosterone in a cohort of 1072 men." Eur J Endocrinol. 151.2 (2004): 241-9.

Nakhla AM, et al. Human sex hormone-binding globulin gene expression-multiple promoters and complex alternative splicing. BMC Mol Biol. 2009 May 5;10:37.

Nankin HR, Calkins JH. Decreased bioavailable testosterone in aging normal and impotent men. J Clin Endocrinol Metab. 1986 Dec;63(6):1418-20.

Saad F, Gooren L. The role of testosterone in the metabolic syndrome: a review. J Steroid Biochem Mol Biol. 2009 Mar;114(1-2):40-3.

Selby C. Sex hormone binding globulin: origin, function and clinical significance. Ann Clin Biochem. 1990 Nov;27 (Pt 6):532-41.

Vermeulen, A, et al. "A Critical Evaluation of Simple Methods for the Estimation of Free Testosterone in Serum." J Clin Endoc & Metab. 84.10 (1999): 3666-3667.

Zhang Y, et al. Coffee consumption and the incidence of type 2 diabetes in men and women with normal glucose tolerance: The Strong Heart Study. Nutr Metab Cardiovasc Dis. 2011 Jun;21(6):418-23.

Chapter 12:
Estradiol – What You Need to Know

Behl C, et al. "17-beta estradiol protects neurons from oxidative stress-induced cell death in vitro". Biochem. Biophys. Res. Commun. (1995) 216 (2): 473–82.

Collins, P; Rosano, et al. "17 beta-

Estradiol attenuates acetylcholine-induced coronary arterial constriction in women but not men with coronary heart disease". Circulation (1995) 92 (1): 24–30. PMID 7788912.

Ghosh, D, J Griswold, et al. "Structural basis for androgen specificity and oestrogen synthesis in human aromatase.." Nature. 457.7226 (2009): 219-23.

Hill RA, et al. "Estrogen deficiency leads to apoptosis in dopaminergic neurons in the medial preoptic area and arcuate nucleus of male mice". Mol. Cell. Neurosci. (2004) 27 (4): 466–76.

Jankowska EA, et al. Circulating estradiol and mortality in men with systolic chronic heart failure. JAMA. 2009 May 13;301(18):1892-901.

"Klinefelter Syndrome". Health Information. National Institute of Health and Human Development. 2007-02-19. Retrieved 2007-03-24.

Kronenberg HM, et al. Williams Textbook of Endocrinology. Philadelphia, PA: Elsevier; 2008.

Warnock JK, et al. "Combined esterified estrogens and methyltestosterone versus esterified estrogens alone in the treatment of loss of sexual interest in surgically menopausal women". Menopause (2005) 12 (4): 359–60.

http://www.edenics.net/english-word-origins.aspx?word=ESTROGEN

Chapter 13:
Cholesterol – Testosterone Fuel

Brown MS and Goldstein JL (1986) A receptor-mediated pathway for cholesterol homeostasis. Science 232:34-47 Cordain, L. The Paleo Answer. John Wiley & Sons, Inc. Hoboken, New Jersey. 2012

Hussain MM. "Review Article: A proposed model for the assembly of chylomicrons"; Arterosclerosis; Vol. 148; 2000; pages 1-15.

Le NA, Walter MF. The role of hypertriglyceridemia in atherosclerosis. Curr Atheroscler Rep 2007; 9:110-5.

Nelson, D. L.; Cox, M. M. "Lehninger, Principles of Biochemistry" 3rd Ed. Worth Publishing: New York, 2000.

Todd J. Anderson, M.D., et al. The Effect of Cholesterol-Lowering and Antioxidant Therapy on Endothelium-Dependent Coronary Vasomotion. N Engl J Med 1995; 332:488-493.

Toth, Peter. "The "Good Cholesterol" High-Density Lipoprotein". Circulation (2005) 111 (5): e89-e91. Retrieved 2 June 2011.

Turhan S, et al. The association between androgen levels and premature coronary artery disease in men. Joint WHO/FAO expert consultation.. Diet, Nutrition and the Prevention of Chronic Diseases (PDF). Geneva: World Health Organization. (2003) Pages 55–56.

"Your Triglyceride Level". What Your Cholesterol Levels Mean. American Heart Association. Retrieved 2009-05-22. http://www.thecholesteroltruth.com/low-cholesterol-diet-myths-debunked

Chapter 14:
The Truth about Statins

Aberg F, et al. Distribution and redox state of ubiquinones in rat and human tissues. Arch Biochem Biophys. 1992 Jun;295(2):230-4.

Abramson J, Wright J (2007). "Are lipid-lowering guidelines evidence-based?". Lancet 369 (9557): 168–9.

ClinicalTrials.gov NCT00976131 Study of CoQ10 During One Cycle of Doxorubicin Treatment for Breast Cancer. http://www.clinicaltrials.gov/show/NCT00976131"Doing Things Differently", Pfizer 2008 Annual Review, April 23, 2009, p. 15.

Devaraj , Jialal et al. Plant Sterol Fortified Orange Juice Effectively Lowers Choleserol Levels in Mildly Hypercholesterolemic Healthy Individuals. Arterioscler. Thromb. Vasc. Biol 2004;24;25-28

Katzung, Bertram G. Basic and clinical pharmacology. New York: McGraw-Hill Medical Publishing Division. 2006.Kunin, RA. West J Med. 1989 August; 151(2): 208.

Law MR, et al. Quantifying effect of statins on low density lipoprotein cholesterol, ischaemic heart disease, and stroke: systematic review and meta-analysis. BMJ.

2003 Jun 28;326(7404):1423.

Mattson, Grundy et al. Optimising the Effect of Plant Sterols on Cholesterol Absorption in Man. Am J Clin Nutr 1982 Apr;35(4).

Molyneux SL, et al. "Coenzyme Q10: an independent predictor of mortality in chronic heart failure". J. Am. Coll. Cardiol. (October 2008) 52 (18): 1435–41.

Mortensen SA, et al. Long-term coenzyme Q10 therapy: a major advance in the management of resistant myocardial failure.

National Cholesterol Education Program. Third Report of the National Cholesterol Education Program (NCEP) Expert Panel on Detection, Evaluation, and Treatment of High Blood Cholesterol in Adults (Adult Treatment Panel III): Executive Summary. Bethesda, MD: National Institutes of Health. National Heart, Lung, and Blood Institute. 2001. pp. 40. NIH Publication No. 01-3670.

Null, G, et al. Death By Medicine. Life Extension Magazine Report. Aug., 2006.

Okamoto T, et al T. Human serum ubiquinol-10 levels and relationship to serum lipids. Int J Vitam Nutr Res. 1989;59(3):288-92.

Pravst, Igor; Zmitek, Katja; Zmitek. "Coenzyme Q10 Contents in Foods and Fortification Strategies". Critical Reviews in Food Science and Nutrition (2010) 50 (4): 269–80.

Ray KK, et al. Statins and all-cause mortality in high-risk primary prevention: a meta-analysis of 11 randomized controlled trials involving 65,229 participants. Arch Intern Med. 2010 Jun 28;170(12):1024-31.

Shindo Y, et al. Enzymic and non-enzymic antioxidants in epidermis and dermis of human skin. J Invest Dermatol. 1994 Jan;102(1):122-4.

Simons, J. "The $10 billion pill", Fortune magazine, January 20, 2003.

Sweetman, SC. et al. "Cardiovascular drugs". Martindale: the complete drug reference (36th ed.). London: Pharmaceutical Press. 2009, pp. 1155–434.

Taylor F, et al. Statins for the primary prevention of cardiovascular disease. Cochrane Database Syst Rev. 2011 Jan 19;(1):CD004816.

Tonelli M, et al. Alberta Kidney Disease Network. CMAJ. 2011 Nov 8;183(16):E1189-202. Epub 2011 Oct 11. Efficacy of statins for primary prevention in people at low cardiovascular risk: a meta-analysis.

Tracy, MJ. "Ch. 4: Coenzyme Q10 (Ubiquinone, Ubidecarenone)". Dietary supplements: toxicology and clinical pharmacology. Humana Press. (2003) pp. 53–85. ISBN 978-1-58829-014-4. US National Center for Health Statistics. National Vital Statistics Report, vol. 51, no. 5, March 14, 2003.

Vanstone, Raeini-Sarjaz et al. Unesterified Plant Sterols and Stanols Lower LDL-cholesterol Concentrations Equivalently in Hypercholesterolemic Persons. Am J Nutr. 2002 Dec;76(8):1272-8

Weber, C; Bysted, A; Hilmer, G. "The coenzyme Q10 content of the average Danish diet". Int J Vitam Nutr Res (1997) 67 (2): 123–9.

http://www.mayoclinic.com/health/statin-side-effects/MY00205

http://sytrinol.net/

http://www.nhs.uk/news/2010/05May/Pages/side-effects-of-statins-studied.aspx

http://medicationsense.com/articles/jan_dec_08/statin_sidefects012108.html

http://www.websters-online-dictionary.org/definitions/snake+oil

Chapter 15:
The Truth about ED Drugs

Aversa A, et al. Effects of vardenafil administration on intravaginal ejaculatory latency time in men with lifelong premature ejaculation. International Journal of Impotence Research (2009) 21, 221–227

Billups KL, et al. Erectile Dysfunction Is a Marker for Cardiovascular Disease: Results of the Minority Health Institute Expert Advisory Panel. The Journal of Sexual Medicine. Volume 2 Issue 1 Page 40 - January 2005

Boolell M, et al. Sildenafil: an orally active type 5 cyclic GMP-specific phosphodiesterase inhibitor for the treatment of penile erectile dysfunction. Int J Impot Res. 1996 Jun;8(2):47-52

Daugan, A, et al. "The discovery of tadalafil: a novel and highly selective PDE5 inhibitor. 1: 5,6,11,11a-tetrahydro-1H-imidazo[1',5':1,6]pyrido[3,4-b]indole-1,3(2H)-dione analogues". (October 9, 2003) J Med Chem. 2003 Oct 9;46(21):4525-32.

"FDA Announces Revisions to Labels for Cialis, Levitra and Viagra". Food and Drug Administration. 2007-10-18.

Johannes CB, et al. Incidence of erectile dysfunction in men 40 to 69 years old: longitudinal results from the Massachusetts male aging study. Journal of Urology 2000 Feb;163(2):460-3

Keith A. "The economics of Viagra" (PDF). Health Aff (Millwood) 19 (2): 147–57. (2000).

Loyd, L. "Two Pills Look to Topple Viagra's Reign in Market; Levitra Expects Approval Next Month, Cialis Later This Year". The Philadelphia Inquirer: p. E01 (July 6, 2003).

McCarthy, S. "First they tried to play it safe; Ads for erectile dysfunction drug Cialis bared all - including a scary potential side effect. It was risky but it has paid off". The Globe and Mail: p. B4. (March 5, 2005).

Nurnberg HG, et al. "Recreational use and misuse of phosphodiesterase 5 inhibitors". Romanelli Journal of the American Medical Association-- Treatment of antidepressant-associated sexual dysfunction with sildenafil: a randomized controlled trial. Journal of the American Pharmacists Association (2005). 45 (1): 63–75.

Parker-Pope T. Viagra Is Misunderstood Despite Name Recognition. The Wall Street Journal online. Nov, 11, 2002.

Stimmel GL, Gutierrez MA. Counseling Patients About Sexual Issues. Pharmacotherapy. 2006;26(11):1608-1615.

Vardi M, Nini A. Phosphodiesterase inhibitors for erectile dysfunction in patients with diabetes mellitus. Cochrane Database Syst Rev. 2007 Jan 24;(1):CD002187.

http://health.msn.com/health-topics/sexual-health/mens-sexual-health/erection-problems-erectile-dysfunction-114

http://www.fda.gov/NewsEvents/Newsroom/PressAnnouncements/ucm274642.htm

http://www.fda.gov/NewsEvents/Newsroom/PressAnnouncements/2007/ucm109012.htm

http://www.pharmpro.com/News/Feeds/2010/06/pharmaceutical-companies-bayer-new-erectile-dysfunction-treatment-staxyn-approve/

Chapter 16:
Testosterone Enhancing Nutrition – Fat Fuel

Beare-Rogers, J.; Dieffenbacher, A.; Holm, J.V. "Lexicon of lipid nutrition (IUPAC Technical Report)". Pure and Applied Chemistry (2001) 73 (4): 685–744.

Binkoski AE, et al. Balance of unsaturated fatty acids is important to a cholesterol-lowering diet: comparison of mid-oleic sunflower oil and olive oil on cardiovascular disease risk factors. J Am Diet Assoc. 2005 Jul;105(7):1080-6.

Clark, M (2011-03-01). "Once a Villain, Coconut Oil Charms the Health Food World". The New York Times. Retrieved 2011-03-02.

David J. Anneken, et al. "Fatty Acids" in Ullmann's Encyclopedia of Industrial Chemistry 2006, Wiley-VCH, Weinheim.

Feinberg School > Nutrition > Nutrition Fact Sheet: Lipids Northwestern University http://nuinfo-proto4.northwestern.edu/nutrition/factsheets/lipids.html

French MA, Sundram K, Clandinin MT. "Cholesterolaemic effect of palmitic acid in relation to other dietary fatty acids". Asia Pacific journal of clinical nutrition. (2002) 11 Suppl 7 (s7): S401–7.

Gosline, Anna (2006-06-12). "Why fast foods are bad, even in moderation". New

Scientist. Retrieved 2007-01-09.

Hayes, K.C. Dietary fat and blood lipids. (May 2005). http://people.brandeis.edu/~kchayes/bginfo.html

Hunter JE, Zhang J, Kris-Etherton PM. Cardiovascular disease risk of dietary stearic acid compared with trans, other saturated, and unsaturated fatty acids: a systematic review. Am J Clin Nutr. 2010 Jan;91(1):46-63. Epub 2009 Nov 25.

Jorge C, wt al. (April 1, 2006). "A prospective study of blood trans fatty acid levels and risk of prostate cancer". Proc. Amer. Assoc. Cancer Res. (American Association for Cancer Research) 47 (1): 943. Retrieved 2007-01-09.

"Lexicon of lipid nutrition (IUPAC Technical Report)". Pure and Applied Chemistry 73 (4): 685–744. 2001.

Lopez-Garcia, et al. "Consumption of Trans Fatty Acids Is Related to Plasma Biomarkers of Inflammation and Endothelial Dysfunction". The Journal of Nutrition (March 1, 2005) 135 (3): 562–566.

Mahfouz M. "Effect of dietary trans fatty acids on the delta 5, delta 6 and delta 9 desaturases of rat liver microsomes in vivo". Acta biologica et medica germanica (1981) 40 (12): 1699–1705.

Mensink RP, et al. "Effects of dietary fatty acids and carbohydrates on the ratio of serum total to HDL cholesterol and on serum lipids and apolipoproteins: a meta-analysis of 60 controlled trials". American Journal of Clinical Nutrition (May 2003) 77 (5): 1146–1155.

Mozaffarian D, et al. "Trans Fatty Acids and Cardiovascular Disease". New England Journal of Medicine (April 13, 2006) 354 (15): 1601–1613.

Naghii MR, et al. Effect of combination therapy of Fatty acids, calcium, vitamin d and boron with regular physical activity on cardiovascular risk factors in rat. J Oleo Sci. 2012;61(2):103-11.

"National nutrient database for standard reference, release 23". United States Department of Agriculture, Agricultural Research Service. 2011. http://www.nal.usda.gov/fnic/foodcomp/search/

Nevin KG, Rajamohan T. Source Wet and dry extraction of coconut oil: impact on lipid metabolic and antioxidant status in cholesterol coadministered rats. Can J Physiol Pharmacol. 2009 Aug;87(8):610-6.

Patterson RE, et al. "Marine Fatty Acid Intake is Associated with Breast Cancer Prognosis". The Journal of Nutrition (2010) 141 (2): 201–206.

Roan, Shari (28 January 2011). "Trans fats and saturated fats could contribute to depression". Sydney Morning Herald. Retrieved 8 February 2011.

Trans Fat Task Force (June 2006). TRANSforming the Food Supply (Appendix 9iii). Retrieved 2007-01-09. [dead link] (Consultation on the health implications of alternatives to trans fatty acids: Summary of Responses from Experts).

http://www.organicfacts.net/organic-oils/organic-coconut-oil/health-benefits-of-coconut-oil.html

http://www.globalsecurity.org/military/systems/munitions/napalm.htm

http://www.mens-fitness-and-health.com/Testosterone-Diet.html

http://www.peaktestosterone.com/Testosterone_Diet.aspx

Chapter 17:
Testosterone Enhancing Nutrition – Protein Fuel

Bouthegourd JC, et al. A preexercise alpha-lactalbumin-enriched whey protein meal preserves lipid oxidation and decreases adiposity in rats. Am J Physiol Endorrinol Metab. 2002 Sep;283(3):E565-72.

Combaret L, et al. Human Nutrition Research Centre of Clermont-Ferrand. "A leucine-supplemented diet restores the defective postprandial inhibition of proteasome-dependent proteolysis in aged rat skeletal muscle". J Physiol. 2005 Dec 1;569(Pt 2):489-99.

Cordain, L. The Paleo Answer. John Wiley & Sons, Inc. Hoboken, New Jersey. 2012 da Luz CR, et al. Potential therapeutic effects of branched-chain amino acids supplementation on resistance exercise-based muscle damage in humans. J Int Soc Sports Nutr. 2011 Dec 14;8:23.

Genton L, Melzer K, Pichard C. Energy and macronutrient requirements for physical fitness in exercising subjects. Clin Nutr. 2010 Aug;29(4):413-23. Epub 2010 Mar 2

De Bandt JP, Cynober L, Branched-Chain Amino Acids: Metabolism, Physiological Function, and Application: Session IV Therapeutic Use of Branched-Chain Amino Acids in Burn, Trauma, and Sepsis1,2 American Society for Nutrition J. Nutr. 136:308S-313S, January 2006

Foegeding, EA; et al. "Advances in modifying and understanding whey protein functionality". Trends in Food Science & Technology (2002) 13 (5): 151–9

Ha E, Zemel MB. "Functional properties of whey, whey components, and essential amino acids: mechanisms underlying health benefits for active people (review)". J. Nutr. Biochem. (May 2003) 14 (5): 251–8.

Hakkak R, et al. "Dietary whey protein protects against azoxymethane-induced colon tumors in male rats". Cancer Epidemiol. Biomarkers Prev. (May 2001) 10 (5): 555–8. PMID 11352868.

Hermann, Janice R.. "Protein and the Body". Oklahoma Cooperative Extension Service, Division of Agricultural Sciences and Natural Resources • Oklahoma State University: Retrieved February 12, 2012.

Krissansen GW. "Emerging health properties of whey proteins and their clinical implications". J Am Coll Nutr (December 2007) 26 (6): 713S–23S.

Laferrère B, Reilly D, Arias S. Differential Metabolic Impact of Gastric Bypass Surgery Versus Dietary Intervention in Obese Diabetic Subjects Despite Identical Weight Loss. Metabolism, Sci Transl Med 27 April 2011: Vol. 3, Issue 80, p. 80re2 Sci. Transl. Med.

Layman DK. The role of leucine in weight loss diets and glucose homeostasis. J Nutr. 2003 Jan;133(1):261S-267S.

R.H.A. Plimmer & F.G. Hopkins. ed. The chemical composition of the proteins. Monographs on biochemistry. Part I. Analysis (2nd ed.). London: Longmans, Green and Co.. p. 112. Retrieved January 18, 2010.

Longcope C, et al. Diet and Sex Hormone-Binding Globulin. J Clin Endoc & Metab. January 1, 2000 vol. 85 no. 1 293-296

Markus CR, et al. Whey protein rich in alpha-lactalbumin increases the ratio of plasma tryptophan to the sum of the other large neutral amino acids and improves cognitive performance in stress-vulnerable subjects. Am J Clin Nutr. 2002 Jun;75(6):1051-6.

Markus CR, et al. Alpha-lactalbumin improves sleep and morning alertness in participants with mild sleep problems. Am J Clin Nutr. 2005 May;81(5):1026-33.

S.C. Mitchell. "Food Idiosyncrasies: Beetroot and Asparagus". Drug Metabolism and Disposition (2001) 29 (4 Pt 2): 539–534.

Welbourne TC. Increased plasma bicarbonate and growth hormone after an oral glutamine load. Am J Clin Nutr. 1995 May;61(5):1058-61.

http://www.vitamins-supplements.org/amino-acids/branched-chain-amino-acids.php

Chapter 18:
Testosterone Supporting Nutrients

Auborn, KJ, et al. "Lifespan is prolonged in autoimmune-prone (NZB/NZW) F1 mice fed a diet supplemented with indole-3-carbinol". The Journal of nutrition (2003) 133 (11): 3610–3.

Balch, Phyllis A., CNC, Balch, James F., M.D., Prescription for Nutritional Healing, Avery Press, p. 104 (2000).

Berdanier, CD, et al. Handbook of Nutrition and Food. Boca Raton, Florida: CRC Press. 2007. ISBN 0849392187.

Chacón de Popovici G. La importancia de Lepidium peruvianum ("Maca") en la alimentacion y salud del ser humano y animal 2,000 anos antes y despues del Cristo y en el siglo XXI. (1997) Lima:

Servicios Gráficos "ROMERO".

Chan, KL, et al. "The effect of Eurycoma longifolia on sperm quality of male rats". Natural product communications (2009) 4 (10): 1331–6.

Chen S, Kao YC, Laughton CA. Binding characteristics of aromatase inhibitors and phytoestrogens to human aromatase. J Steroid Biochem Mol Biol 1997 Apr;61(3-6):107-15).

Clark LC, et al. Effects of selenium supplementation for cancer prevention in patients with carcinoma of the skin. A randomized controlled trial. Nutritional Prevention of Cancer Study Group. JAMA. 1996 Dec 25;276(24):1957-63.

Cyranoski, D. "Malaysian researchers bet big on home-grown Viagra". Nature Medicine (2005) 11 (9): 912.

Dording CM, et al. "A double-blind, randomized, pilot dose-finding study of maca root (L. meyenii) for the management of SSRI-induced sexual dysfunction". CNS Neurosci Ther (December 2009) 14 (3): 182–91.

Gonzales GF, et al. "Effect of Lepidium meyenii (maca) on sexual desire and its absent relationship with serum testosterone levels in adult healthy men". Andrologia (2002) 34 (6): 367–72.

Gonzales GF, et al. "Lepidium meyenii (maca) improved semen parameters in adult men". Asian Journal of Andrology (2001) 3 (4): 301–3. PMID 11753476.

Gonzales GF, et al. "Lepidium meyenii (Maca): a plant from the highlands of Peru--from tradition to science". Forsch Komplementmed 16 (6): 373–80.

Gonzales GF, et al. "Effect of Lepidium meyenii (Maca), a root with aphrodisiac and fertility-enhancing properties, on serum reproductive hormone levels in adult healthy men". J Endocrinol. (Jan 2003) 176 (1): 163–8.

Hambidge, K. M. and Krebs, N. F. "Zinc deficiency: a special challenge". J. Nutr. (2007) 137 (4): 1101–5.

Jeong HG, et al. Inhibition of aromatase activity by flavonoids. Arch Pharm Res 1999 Jun;22(3):309-12.

Kellis JT Jr, Vickery LE. "Inhibition of human estrogen synthetase (aromatase) by flavones". Science (1984) 225 (4666): 1032–4.

Kilham C. Tales from the Medicine Trail: Tracking Down the Health Secrets of Shamans, Herbalists, Mystics, Yogis, and Other Healers. [Emmaus PA]: Rodale Press (2000).

Majeed, M. Use of piperine as a bioavailability enhancer. US Patent 5744161

Matsuoka, K, .et al. Study of Thermodynamic Parameters for Solubilization of Plant Sterol and Stanol in Bile Salt Micelles. Chem. Phys. Lipids 2008, 154, 87-93.

Prasad AS. Zinc deficiency: Has been known of for 40 years but ignored by global health organisations". BMJ. 2003 February 22; 326(7386): 409–410.

Rosen, CA., Bryson, PC. "Indole-3-Carbinol for recurrent respiratory papillomatosis: Long-term results". Journal of Voice (2004) 18 (2): 248–53.

Safarinejad MR. Urtica dioica for treatment of benign prostatic hyperplasia: a prospective, randomized, double-blind, placebo-controlled, crossover study. J Herb Pharmacother.. 2005;5(4):1-11.

Schöttner M, et al. Interaction of lignans with human sex hormone binding globulin (SHBG). " Z Naturforsch [C]". 1997 Nov–Dec;52(11–12):834–43.

Shah, M, et al. "Direct intra-tumoral injection of zinc-acetate halts tumor growth in a xenograft model of prostate cancer". Journal of Experimental and Clinical Cancer Research 28 (84): 84.

Teucher T, et al. Cytokine secretion in whole blood of healthy subjects following oral administration of Urtica dioica L. plant extract. Arzneimittelforschung 1996 Sep;46(9):906–10

Wahab, NA, et al. "The Effect of Eurycoma Longifolia Jack on Spermatogenesis in Estrogen-Treated Rats". (2010). Clinics 65 (1): 93–8.

Westfall R.E., Galactagogue herbs: a qualitative study and review. Canadian

Journal of Midwifery Research and Practice. 2(2):22–27. (2003).

Zheng, BLet al. "Effect of a lipidic extract from Lepidium meyenii on sexual behavior in mice and rats". Urology (2000) 55 (4): 598–602.

http://pubchem.ncbi.nlm.nih.gov/summary/summary.cgi?cid=5318997

http://www.babylon.com/define/108/Indonesian-English-Dictionary.html

http://www.aimforherbs.com/pollenextract.html

http://ods.od.nih.gov/factsheets/selenium/#h2

Chapter 19:
Don't Exercise – Biocize®

Alessio, H.M.; Exercise-induced Oxidative Stress, Med Sci Sports Exerc, (Feb 1993), 25:2, 218–24.

Brsheim, E., et al; "Adrenergic Control of Post-exercise Metabolism," Acta Physiol Scand, 162 (Mar 1998):313–23.

Burke, ER.; Optimal Muscle Recovery, Avery Publishing Group, 1999.

Coggan A.R. et al. "Fat Metabolism During High-Intensity Exercise in Endurance-Trained and Untrained Men," Metabolism 49 (2000):122–8.

Cooper KH. Can stress heal?. Thomas Nelson Inc. (1997) p. 40

Fernández Pastor V.J., et al; "Function of Growth Hormone in the Human Energy Continuum During Physical Exertion," Rev Esp Fisiol, 47 (Dec 1991):223–9.

Fiatarone, M.A., et al; "High-intensity Strength Training in Nonagenerians. Effects on Skeletal Muscle." J of the American Medical Association, 263 (1990):3029–3034.

Harro J., et al; "Association of Depressiveness with Blunted Growth Hormone Response to Maximal Physical Exercise in Young Healthy Men," Psychoneuroendocrinology, 24 (Jul 1999):505–17.

Karlsson J.; Metabolic Adaptations to Exercise: A Review of Potential Beta-adrenoceptor Antagonist Effects, Am J Cardiol, 55 (Apr 1985):48D–58D.

Kent M. Aerobic exercise', Food and Fitness: A Dictionary of Diet and Exercise, Oxford University Press, 1997.

Kraemer W.J. et al. "Effects of Heavy-Resistance Training on Hormonal Response Patterns in Younger and Older Men," J Appl Physiol 87(1999):982–92.

Kraemer W.J., et al; "Endogenous Anabolic Hormonal and Growth Factor Responses to Heavy Resistance Exercise in Males and Females," Int _J Sports Med, 12 (Apr 1991):228–35.

McAuley E.; Mihalko SL; Bane SM; "Exercise and Self-Esteem in Middle-Aged Adults: Multidimensional Relationships and Physical Fitness and Self-Efficacy Influences," J Behav Med, 20 (Feb 1997):67–83.

McCartney, N.A., et al; "Usefulness of Weightlifting Training in Improving Strength and Maximal Power Output in Coronary Artery Disease," Amer J Cardiol, 67 (1991):939.

Pate RR, et al. Physical activity and public health. A recommendation from the Centers for Disease Control and Prevention and the American College of Sports Medicine. JAMA. 1995 Feb 1;273(5):402-7.

Plowman SA , et al. Exercise Physiology for Health, Fitness, and Performance. (June 2007) SLippincott Williams & Wilkins. p. 61

Tabata I, et al. "Effects of moderate-intensity endurance and high-intensity intermittent training on anaerobic capacity and VO2max". Med Sci Sports Exerc (1996) 28 (10): 1327–30.

Tabata I, et al. "Metabolic profile of high intensity intermittent exercises". Med Sci Sports Exerc (March 1997). 29 (3): 390–5.

Zmuda JM, Thompson PD & Winters SJ. Exercise Increases Serum Testosterone and Sex Hormone-Binding Globulin Levels in Older Men. Metabolism. 1996 Aug;45(8):935-9.

Chapter 20:
Booze – Babies and Testosterone

Altura BM, Altura BT. Association of

alcohol in brain injury, headaches, and stroke with brain-tissue and serum levels of ionized magnesium: a review of recent findings and mechanisms of action. Alcohol. 1999 Oct;19(2):119-30.

Badr FM, et al. Suppression of testosterone production by ethyl alcohol. Possible mode of action. Steroids. 1977 Nov;30(5):647-55.

Hannak D, , et al. Acetatex formation after short-term ethanol administration in man. Biol Chem Hoppe Seyler 1985; 366:749–53.

Lundquist F, et al. Ethanol metabolism and production of free acetate in the human liver. J Clin Invest 1962;41:955–61.

Siler, SQ, et al. De novo lipogenesis, lipid kinetics, and whole-body lipid balances in humans after acute alcohol consumption. American Journal of Clinical Nutrition, 70, 928-936, 1999.

Valimaki, MJ, et al. Sex hormones and adrenocortical steroids in men acutely intoxicated with ethanol. Alcohol, 1, 89-93, 1984.

http://umich.academia.edu/SarivanAnders/Papers/990830/Baby_cries_and_nurturance_affect_testosterone_in_men

http://yourlife.usatoday.com/health/medical/menshealth/story/2011-09-13/Fathers-tstosterone-drops-steeply-after-baby-arrives/50384024/1

http://helpguide.org/mental/stress_management_relief_coping.htm

BONUS CHAPTER:
The Unsung Hero – Appreciating Your Better Half

Agarwal R. Antimetastatic efficacy of silibinin: Molecular mechanisms and therapeutic potential against cancer Deep G., Cancer and Metastasis Reviews 2010 29:3 (447-463)

Bick J, Dozier M. Mother's and Ch ildren's Concentrations of Oxytocin Folllowing Close, Physical Interactions with Biological and non-biological Children. Dev Psychobiol (January 2010). 52 (1): 100–107.

Byrne J. Study finds broccoli extract could inhibit breast cancer cells.

Nutraingredients.com. May, 5, 2010

Chiodera P, et al. "Different effects of the serotonergic agonists buspirone and sumatriptan on the posterior pituitary hormonal responses to hypoglycemia in humans". Neuropeptides (April 1996) 30 (2): 187–92.

Dale HH. On some physiological actions of ergot. J. Physiol. (Lond.) (May 1906). 34 (3): 163–206.

du Vigneaud V, Ressler C, Trippett S. "The sequence of amino acids in oxytocin, with a proposal for the structure of oxytocin". J. Biol. Chem. (Dec. 1953). 205 (2): 949–57.

Fewtrell MS, et al. " Randomised, double blind trial of Oxytocin nasal spray in mothers expressing breast milk for preterm infants". Archives of Disease in Childhood. Fetal and Neonatal Edition (May 2006) 91 (3): F169–74.

Genital HPV Infection — CDC Fact Sheet". Centers for Disease Control and Prevention (CDC). April 10, 2008. Retrieved 13 November 2009.

Guastella AJ, Mitchell PB, Dadds MR. "Oxytocin increases gaze to the eye region of human faces". Biological Psychiatry (Jan 2008). 63 (1): 3–5.

Hatcher H., et al. "Curcumin: from ancient medicine to current clinical trials". Cell. Mol. Life Sci. (June 2008).65 (11): 1631–52.

Kendrick KM. The Neurobiology of Social Bonds. British Society for Neuroendocrinology. (2004-01-01) Retrieved 2009-04-13.

Kroll DJ, et al. Milk thistle nomenclature: why it matters in cancer research and pharmacokinetic studies. Integrative Cancer Therapies. (2007) 6: 110-119.

Kuchinskas S. The Chemistry of Connection: How the Oxytocin Response Can Help You Find Trust, Intimacy, and Love. New Harbinger Publications Inc. Oakland CA. 2009. p65

Kutluay SB, et al. "Curcumin inhibits herpes simplex virus immediate-early gene expression by a mechanism independent of p300/CBP histone acetyltransferase activity". Virology (January 2008) 373 (2): 239–47.

Lee HJ, et al. Oxytocin the Great Facilitator of Life. Progress in Neurobiology (June 2009). 88 (2): 127–51.

Mayer L. Peruvian Maca… A New Alternative for Women's Health. Women's Journal. July, 5, 2010.

Marazziti D, et al. A relationship between Oxytocin and anxiety of romantic attachment. Clin Pract Epidemiol Ment Health (2006). 2: 28.

National Center for Complementary and Alternative Medicine. "Milk Thistle". National Institutes of Health. - General information on milk thistle.

O'Callaghan, T. "Thanks Mom". Time Magazine (Time, Inc.). (7, June 2010). Retrieved 2010-06-08.

Ott I, Scott JC. The Action of Infundibulum upon Mammary Secretion. Proc Soc Exp Biol. (1910) p.8:48–49.

Petrovic P, et al. "Oxytocin Attenuates Affective Evaluations of Conditioned Faces and Amygdala Activity". The Journal of Neuroscience (June 2008) 28 (26): 6607–15.

Prakash P, Gupta N. "Therapeutic uses of Ocimum sanctum Linn (Tulsi) with a note on eugenol and its pharmacological actions: A short review". Indian Journal of Physiology and Pharmacology (April 2005) 49 (2): 125–131.

Qingdi Q, et al. "-Elemene, a novel plant-derived antineoplastic agent, increases cisplatin chemosensitivity of lung tumor cells by triggering apoptosis". Oncology Reports (2009) 22: 161–170.

Rahman A, Isenberg DA. "Review Article: Systemic Lupus Erythematosus". N Engl J Med 358 (February 28, 2008).

Rosen CA, Bryson PC. "Indole-3-Carbinol for recurrent respiratory papillomatosis: Long-term results". Journal of Voice (2004) 18 (2): 248–53.

Ross HE, et al. Characterization of the Ixytocin System Regulating Affiliative Behavior in Female Prairie Voles. Neuroscience (Sept. 2009). 162 (4): 892–903.

Schafer EA, Mackenzie K. The action of animal extracts on milk secretion. Proceedings of the Royal Society of London Series B-Containing Papers of a Biological Character. (1911) p.84:16–22.

Singer T, et al. Effects of Oxytocin and Prosocial Behavior on Brain Responses to Direct and Vicariously Experienced Pain. Emotion (December 2008). 8 (6): 781–91.

Ströfer M, et al. "Curcumin decreases survival of Hep3B liver and MCF-7 breast cancer cells: the role of HIF." Strahlenther Onkol. 2011 Jul;187(7):393-400.

The Chemistry of Connection: How the Oxytocin Response Can Help You Find Trust, Intimacy, and Love endocrinology of sexual arousal". The Journal of Endocrinology (Sept. 2005).186 (3): 411–27.

Uvnäs-Moberg K, et al. "Effects of 5-HT agonists, selective for different receptor subtypes, on oxytocin, CCK, gastrin and somatostatin plasma levels in the rat". Neuropharmacology (1996). 35 (11): 1635–40.

Vacek M. What can voles teach us about monogamy? American Scientist online. (May-June, 2002) High on Fidelity.

Zak PJ, Stanton AA, Ahmadi S. Oxytocin Increases Generosity in Humans. PLoS ONE (2007) 2(11): e1128.

http://www.dglucarate.com/Glucarate_Report.pdf

http://www.hindunet.org/faq/fom-serv/cache/19.html

http://www.uni-graz.at/~katzer/engl/Ocim_bas.html

http://bit.ly/xCvDP7

http://bit.ly/qfjWM7

///

Part III

Chapter 21:
The Top 10 Beer Belly Blues Banishers

1) Change Your Attitude

Booth A, et al. Testosterone, and winning and losing in human competition. Horm

Behav. 1989 Dec;23(4):556-71.

Mazur A, Booth A. Testosterone and dominance in men. Behav Brain Sci. (1998), 21 : pp 353-363

McCraty R, et al. The impact of a new emotional self-management program on stress, emotions, heart rate variability, DHEA and cortisol. Integr Physiol Behav Sci. 1998 Apr-Jun;33(2):151-70.

2) Stress-Less
Borghese, C.M., et al. "Cortisol, the Muscle Eater." Brain Res Bull 31 (1993):697–700.

Hansen PA, et al. DHEA protects against visceral obesity and muscle insulin resistance in rats fed a high-fat diet. Am J Physiol. 1997 Nov;273(5 Pt 2):R1704-8.

Jedrzejuk D, et al. Dehydroepiandrosterone replacement in healthy men with age-related decline of DHEA-S: effects on fat distribution, insulin sensitivity and lipid metabolism. Aging Male. 2003 Sep;6(3):151-6.

3) Lose the Grump
Anderson P. Low Testosterone Levels Linked With Higher Risk for Depression. Medscape medical News. March 10, 2008

Murray MT. What the Drug Companies Won't Tell You and Your Doctor Doesn't Know: The Alternative Treatments That May Change Your Life - and the Prescriptions That Could Harm You. Atria Paperbacks, New York, NY. 2010.

Perelman MA. Erectile dysfunction and depression: screening and treatment. Urol Clin North Am. 2011 May;38(2):125-39.

Victoroff J. Saving the Brain, Harper Collins Publishers Inc., New York, NY 2003, p. 85.

4) Sleep Better
Low Testosterone Levels Restrict Deep Sleep. (posted by karinb - May 21, 2010). Thirdage.com.

Penev PD. Association between sleep and morning testosterone levels in older men. Sleep, 2007, 30:427-432

5) Find Your Mojo
Carosa E, et al. Type V phosphodiesterase inhibitor treatments for erectile dysfunction increase testosterone levels. Clin Endocrinol (Oxf). 2004 Sep;61(3):382-6.

Dabbs JM Jr, Mohammed S. Male and female salivary testosterone concentrations before and after sexual activity. Physiology & Behavior, Jul 1992, 52(1):195-197

Graham JM, Desjardins C. Classical conditioning: induction of luteinizing hormone and testosterone secretion in anticipation of sexual activity. Science, Nov 28 1980, 210(4473):1039-1041.

6) Say No to Sugar
Al-Dujaili E, Ashmore S. Effect of Glycaemic index of the diet on salivary cortisol and testosterone levels in females. Endocrine Abstracts (2007) 13 P286

Michaels K. Halt Sugar-Induced Cell Aging. Life Extension Magazine January 2012

Pitteloud N, et al. Increasing insulin resistance is associated with a decrease in Leydig cell testosterone secretion in men. J Clin Endocrinol Metab. 2005 May;90(5):2636-41.

7) Get Some Sun
Cordain L. The Paleo Answer. John Wiley & Sons, Inc. New Jersey, 2012 (pg. 208).

Wehr E, et al. Association of vitamin D status with serum androgen levels in men. Clin Endocrinol (Oxf), 2010 Aug;73(2):243-8. Epub 2009 Dec 29.

8) Lose the Belly
Anderson LA, et al. The effects of androgens and estrogens on preadipocyte proliferation in human adipose tissue: influence of gender and site. J Clin Endocrinol Metab. 2001 Oct;86(10):5045-51.

Gooren L, et al. The metabolic syndrome: when is testosterone treatment warranted. J of Mens Health, Sep 2008, 5(1):S40-S45.

Heidler S, et al. Is the metabolic syndrome an independent risk factor for erectile dysfunction? Jour Urol, 2007 Feb, 177(2):651-4

Vermeulen A. Androgen replacement therapy in the aging male--a critical evaluation. J Clin Endocrinol Metab, 2001 Jun;86(6):2380-90.

Zumoff B, et al. Plasma free and nonsex-hormone-binding-globulin-bound testosterone are decreased in obese men in proportion to their degree of obesity. Jour Clin Endocrin Metab 1990 Oct,71(4):929-31

9) Don't Overtrain

Gleeson M. Immune function in sport and exercise. J Appl Physiol. 2007 Aug;103(2):693-9. Epub 2007 Feb 15.

MacKinnon LT. Special feature for the Olympics: effects of exercise on the immune system: overtraining effects on immunity and performance in athletes. Immunol Cell Biol. 2000 Oct;78(5):502-9.

10) Up Your BCAAs

Sharp CP, Pearson DR. Amino Acid Supplements and Recovery from High-Intensity Resistance Training. J Strength Cond Res, 2010; 24(4): 1125-1130

For more information please visit
www.UltimateMaleSolution.com

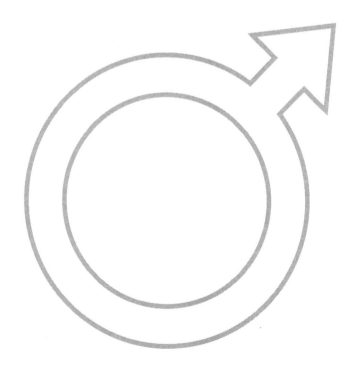